THE BREATHING
DISORDERS
SOURCEBOOK

Also by Francis V. Adams:
The Asthma Sourcebook

THE BREATHING DISORDERS SOURCEBOOK

by
Francis V. Adams, M.D.

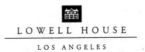

LOWELL HOUSE

LOS ANGELES

NTC/Contemporary Publishing Group

Library of Congress Cataloging in Publication Data

Adams, Fráncis V.
    The breathing disorders sourcebook / by Francis V. Adams.
        p.   cm.
    ISBN 0-7373-0006-X
    1. Respiratory organs—Diseases.   2. Lungs—Diseases, Obstructive.
I. Title.
    [DNLM: 1. Respiratory Tract Diseases.   WF 140A212b 1998]
    RC731.A32   1998
    616.2—dc21
                                                                        98-27806
                                                                          CIP

Published by Lowell House, a division of NTC/Contemporary Publishing Group, Inc.
4255 West Touhy Avenue, Lincolnwood, Illinois 60646-1975, U.S.A.

Requests for such permissions should be addressed to:
Lowell House
2020 Avenue of the Stars, Suite 300
Los Angeles, CA 90067

Design by Susan H. Hartman

Printed and bound in the United States of America
International Standard Book Number: 0-7373-0006-X
10 9 8 7 6 5 4 3 2

This book is for my mother, Rose,
and in memory of my father,
Dr. Vincent J. Adams.

CONTENTS

BIBLIOGRAPHY

APPENDIX:
FINDING OUT MORE

GLOSSARY

INDEX

ILLUSTRATIONS

TABLES

INTRODUCTION

B reathing is essential for life. With each breath, the lung functions to provide oxygen as the fuel for metabolism and to excrete carbon dioxide, which is formed as a waste product. Since the body has a limited capacity to store oxygen and carbon dioxide, a continuous exchange of these gases with the environment must occur to preserve life.

The simple act of breathing involves a complex interaction between body sensors and the brain, producing a nerve impulse that is transmitted to the respiratory muscles, which move the lungs. Abnormalities at any point in this sequence, from the nervous system to muscle to lung, may produce a breathing disorder. Distress signals from the lung and other organs, as well as increased demands for exertion, will produce the disturbing sensation of shortness of breath.

Breathing disorders produce a major component of health disease worldwide and are attracting greater attention. One reason for this is the increased awareness of a relationship between the environment and lung disease. A direct connection has already been established between the levels of air pollution and an increased incidence of lung diseases such as asthma. This knowledge follows several decades of the detailing of the cause-and-effect relationship between cigarette smoking and lung disease. The fact that these breathing disorders are preventable has fueled interest in stricter government regulation of smoking and the environment.

Almost 335,000 Americans die of lung disease each year, according to the American Lung Association. Breathing disorders are responsible for one in seven deaths in the United States. Lung disease is the third leading cause of death in this country. While the death rate from the number one and two causes—heart disease and cancer—has decreased, the death rate for lung disease has increased. Between 1979 and 1994, the death rate due to lung disease increased by nearly 19 percent.

Breathing disorders attack all ages and races. Thirty-one percent of infant deaths in 1994 were attributed to lung disease. Among African Americans the lung disease rate is 16.3 percent higher than for Caucasians. In the elderly and individuals with cancer and AIDS, conditions in which there are lowered immune defenses, life-threatening lung infections often develop.

Breathing disorders do more than kill. Much of lung disease is chronic, producing a continuous struggle to breathe. It is estimated that more than thirty million Americans have chronic lung disease, including fourteen million asthmatics and sixteen million individuals with smoking-related chronic obstructive pulmonary disease. Chronic lung disease produces the greatest amount of disability among workers in the United States. It is also expensive, costing the American economy $33.4 billion in direct health-care expenditures each year, plus indirect costs of more than $51 billion, totaling more than $85 billion.

It is my belief that an informed patient is a healthier patient. This book is intended to provide general information on breathing disorders, improving awareness, and to stimulate patient-physician interaction. In this era of managed medical care, access to physicians and especially medical specialists has been limited. The informed patient is more likely to receive the appropriate care.

After the publication of *The Asthma Sourcebook,* many individuals urged me to write about other breathing disorders. This book is the culmination of their suggestions. I am unable, however, to include every known breathing disorder or to discuss all aspects of treatment of these diseases. Hopefully, this book will serve as a starting point for those interested in chest diseases. The appendix lists many additional resources that the reader may want to explore. As our knowledge of lung function and disease increases, I continue to be fascinated by the intricate workings of the respiratory system. I hope that the reader will also be intrigued by this amazing system.

As in many areas of medicine, the diagnosis and treatment of breathing disorders is not devoid of controversy. The opinions expressed in this book are drawn from my own experience in chest medicine, which now spans nearly twenty-five years.

I could not have written this book without the help and support of many individuals. I can only name a few. The medical illustrations were done by my wife, Laurel H. Adams. To write this book, Laurie also allowed me to take the time from the daily hours that we normally spend together. I know of no greater gift than this. Mary Kane provided invaluable research, materials, and suggestions that have been used in this manuscript. A great deal of the information provided in the appendix comes from Ms. Kane's contribution, which included endless hours exploring the Internet. I also wish to thank my editor, Bud Sperry, of Lowell House, who was receptive to the idea of this project and guided me through to publication.

You still shall live (such virtue hath my pen)
Where breath most breathes, even in the mouths of men.

William Shakespeare, *Sonnet lxxxi.*

1

How We Breathe

One of the most common and challenging problems that a pulmonologist is called upon to treat is respiratory failure. In this situation, the body has failed to supply adequate amounts of oxygen and to excrete carbon dioxide. If not corrected, this condition will prove fatal. With each patient it is best to try to determine what went wrong with the respiratory system, while at the same time attempting to correct oxygen and carbon dioxide levels. This chapter will explore the normal mechanisms that produce breathing. This information will form the basis for the understanding of how the respiratory system may fail.

As a first-year fellow in pulmonary disease at Bellevue Hospital in 1973, I was assigned to a rotation in the intensive care unit. A large percentage of the patients in the ICU had suffered respiratory failure, and many were being supported by mechanical respirators. One of my daily tasks was to measure the breathing function of the patients on respirators to see if they could again breathe on their own. I would attach a small flowmeter called a Wright spirometer to the end of the breathing tube that had been inserted into the patient's windpipe and perform several breathing measurements. When the patient's performance reached a certain level, the breathing tube was removed. One patient I saw daily in this capacity was a young woman who had been hospitalized with a rare neurologic disease called Guillain-Barré syndrome. She had always been entirely well except for a recent viral illness but was hospitalized with severe muscle weakness that had started in her legs and progressed to involve her breathing muscles. Fortunately, this syndrome usually has a good outcome, but recovery is slow and she had been on a mechanical respirator for several weeks. Unable to speak due to the tube in her throat, she would communicate with me with her eyes or with a brief, scribbled note. I often told her that we would have a long conversation when the tube was removed. When her bedside measurements revealed sufficient recovery of her breathing muscles and the breathing tube had been removed, I went by to see her. As soon as she saw me she whispered, "I can breathe."

THE NERVOUS SYSTEM

A brief overview of the human nervous system is necessary for the understanding of how we breathe. The nervous system is divided into the "central" structures of the brain and spinal cord and the peripheral nerve structures distributed throughout the body.

Nerve impulses travel from the brain and spinal cord through electrical and chemical means. Input signals from body receptors that sense temperature, pressure, and pain travel in the opposite direction. Nervous system actions are often termed voluntary or automatic. An example of voluntary activity would be the brain signal that directs the muscles of the arm to move. Breathing is an example of an automatic function, but it may also be voluntary.

The Autonomic Nervous System

A major subdivision of the peripheral nervous system is called the autonomic nervous system, which is responsible for the involuntary control of major body functions. It is divided into a parasympathetic and a sympathetic branch. These systems extend throughout the body but are important in respiratory function. Think of these two systems as balancing each other. For example, stimulating the parasympathetic system causes the bronchial tubes to constrict, while stimulating the sympathetic nervous system produces the opposite reaction (dilatation).

The effects produced through the nerve pathways are mediated by chemicals called neurotransmitters. In the parasympathetic nervous system, the neurotransmitter is a substance known as acetylcholine. Medications that mimic the effects of this substance are called cholinergic agents. In the sympathetic nervous system the neurotransmitter is a substance known as epinephrine (adrenaline). Medications that mimic the effects of adrenaline are called adrenergic agents.

Receptors

Neurotransmitters work on protein substances on the surface of cells to produce specific effects. These substances are called receptors because they respond only to certain chemicals. In the autonomic nervous system, these receptors are termed alpha and beta. In general, alpha receptors excite, and beta receptors usually inhibit or relax.

THE BRAIN CENTER: CONTROLLER NEURONS

The respiratory system is equipped with multiple nerve centers, which act as sensors that monitor the chemistry of the blood (chemoreceptors) and the action of the lung and chest muscles (mechanoreceptors). These sensors, or receptors, send nerve signals to nerve cells (neurons) in the brain to control breathing.

These controllers are groups of neurons located in regions of the brain called the brain stem. The brain stem is located between the cortex of the brain and the spinal cord. The two centers for the control of breathing are located within portions of the brain stem called the pons and the medulla. The neurons in these centers have connections, or synapses, with the endings of nerves that originate in sensors in the neck and chest. Certain neurons appear to be responsible for breathing in, or inspiration, and others for breathing out, or expiration. The nervous system's control of breathing is illustrated in Fig. 1.1.

Ondine's Curse

The knowledge of the existence of neurons that automatically control breathing has come in part from work with stroke patients. As a medical student at Cornell, I was taught by Dr. Fred Plum, one of medicine's most distinguished neurologists. Making rounds with Plum was a unique experience for medical students, as he would pose questions for each of us. It was rare for anyone to have the correct answer. It always seemed that I had the answer for the student ahead and behind me but never for the question meant specifically for me. One such question concerned a patient with "Ondine's curse." Ondine was a water nymph portrayed in Jean Giraudoux's adaptation of the German legend called *Ondine*. Betrayed by the unfaithful knight Hans, she took away his automatic function of breathing, and he slept until he died.

A stroke is an injury to the blood supply to the brain, often occurring because of a blockage of a small artery. The neurons that are dependent on the blocked vessel for oxygen die or are injured as a result of the stroke. Plum and other neurologists observed that stroke patients with injuries to certain portions of the medulla may lose their automatic control of breathing and suffer Ondine's curse. A striking feature of these patients is the preservation of the voluntary ability to control breathing.

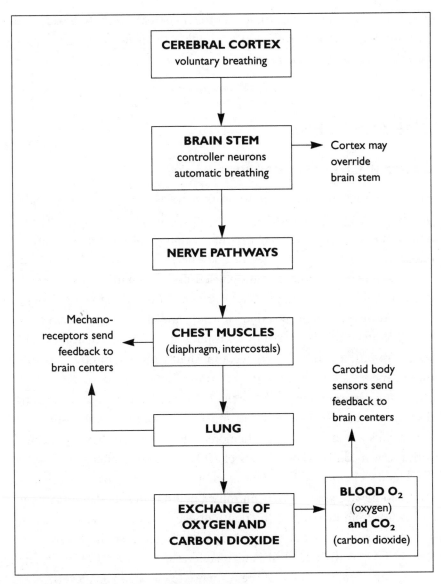

FIG. 1.1 THE CONTROL OF BREATHING.

If asked to breathe deeply, the patient can decrease carbon dioxide and increase oxygen blood levels, but at all other times he or she must have the support of a mechanical respirator.

THE SENSORS

Central Chemoreceptors

Breathing can be maintained voluntarily, as well as automatically through nerve pathways that originate in the brain stem. A remarkable and complex system maintains normal amounts of oxygen and carbon dioxide in the face of changes in body needs, as well as the environment. Through the input of multiple sensors, the controlling brain cells can make almost instantaneous adjustments in breathing, with changes in activity, nourishment, position, altitude, and sleep. This system must also coordinate the function of the respiratory muscles, which move the lungs. All of this must also be accomplished with a minimum expenditure of energy so that breathing is effortless.

In the same portion of the brain stem that contains the controlling neurons are brain cells which are sensitive to levels of carbon dioxide. These cells are called central chemoreceptors because they are located within the medulla. When levels of CO_2 increase, a change occurs in the blood's chemistry. The central chemoreceptors sense this change and send nerve signals to the controlling neurons to stimulate breathing. The result is an increase in the depth of each breath. If the signals persist, the rate or frequency of breathing will also increase. In this way, the level of CO_2 is decreased. It is estimated that the central chemoreceptors account for 70 percent of the response to elevated CO_2 levels.

CRIB DEATH: A MISSING NEUROTRANSMITTER?

Crib death, or sudden infant death syndrome (SIDS), accounts for half of the deaths of infants two to four months old. Recent research has found that SIDS victims have less neurotransmitters present in the controller neurons located in the brain stem. This suggests that as carbon dioxide levels rise and oxygen levels fall during sleep, the brains of certain babies do not receive the signal to alter their breathing to adjust for the change.

Peripheral Chemoreceptors

Sensors located in the neck and chest are called peripheral chemoreceptors and are responsible for the remaining 30 percent of the breathing response to elevated levels of carbon dioxide. One of the most important sensors is located near the carotid artery, a major neck artery, and is called the carotid body. This sensor is important and unique because it is also sensitive to reductions in blood oxygen levels. Changes in oxygen levels produce nerve signals that are transmitted to the controller neurons in the brain stem, resulting in an increase in the depth and rate of breathing. The carotid body is sensitive to even mild changes in oxygen levels and will alert the controlling neurons in the brain to even slight changes.

Research has demonstrated that sensitivity to CO_2 levels varies from person to person. In some individuals, there may be a reduced response to elevations of CO_2. In this situation, the action of the carotid body to stimulate breathing is important and potentially lifesaving.

Respiratory Mechanoreceptors

Sensors, called mechanoreceptors, located throughout the respiratory system, respond to stretch, motion, and tension. These sensors provide the controller brain cells feedback on the mechanical act of breathing. These receptors are located in the lung's air passages, which are called bronchi, as well as in the lung itself. They are involved in the lung's response to illnesses that affect expansion or produce lung congestion or irritation in the air passages. One example is the response of the lung receptors to the inhalation of a noxious gas. When a toxic gas, such as chlorine, is inhaled, the irritant receptors act within seconds to send to the brain signals that produce a protective cough and rapid shallow breathing, which reduce penetration of the noxious fumes.

Additional Receptors

Sensors are also located in the structures that make up the chest wall, which shields the lungs. The chest wall consists of the rib cage, supporting tendons, and breathing muscles that surround and support the lungs. Receptors in this structure's joints, muscles, and tendons provide input to the brain on the movement produced by the respiratory muscles. One of the most important respiratory muscles is the diaphragm, which is largely responsible for inspiration. The diaphragm is a large dome-shaped muscle that separates the lungs from the abdomen and moves up and down with each breath. There is a right and left portion of the diaphragm, which correspond to each lung. The right diaphragm is normally positioned slightly higher than the left.

INTEGRATING THE SIGNALS

In addition to the noted sensors, receptors in the circulatory system—which includes the heart and blood vessels, body temperature centers, and muscles of the arms and legs—also provide signals to the brain's controller neurons. The integration of these multiple inputs provides coordination of respiratory muscles during speech, swallowing, singing, and exercise. These multiple inputs ensure that breathing will be automatically maintained when disease may affect one pathway or when there is decreased consciousness, as in sleep.

When conflict between signals and demands occurs, however, the result is shortness of breath, one of the most common symptoms of chest disease.

Automatic but Also Voluntary

In addition to the automatic control of breathing, a voluntary system exists. The nerve signals for voluntary control of breathing originate in the area of the brain known as the cerebral cortex. Common examples of this voluntary control include holding your breath, speaking, and laughing. During these activities, the voluntary nerve signals override the automatic ones. In addition, the nerve signals to the breathing muscles from the voluntary brain centers travel over different pathways from those originating from the automatic centers.

THE RESPIRATORY SYSTEM

In the first half of the Earth's existence, oxygen (O_2) was present in minute amounts. Approximately two billion years ago, simple life-forms evolved the ability to use O_2 as fuel for metabolism. Carbon dioxide (CO_2) is the end point of this metabolism. The lung's primary function is to exchange O_2 and CO_2 between air that is inspired and blood that circulates throughout the body. In order for this gas exchange to occur efficiently, a large amount of blood must be spread thinly across a huge surface that is in communication with the air. This unique structure is the human lung.

THE NORMAL LUNG

The right and left lungs are attached to the windpipe, or trachea, which begins below the voice box, or larynx. The right lung is slightly larger than the left and has three lobes or divisions; the left has two. The windpipe divides into a right and left channel, called the main stem bronchus. The bronchial tubes are hollow branching air passages, and the entire bronchial system resembles a great oak tree, with its trunk represented by the windpipe. (See Fig. 1.2.) The smallest air passages are called bronchioles, and they end by opening into tiny air sacs, called alveoli. Within the walls of the alveoli are small blood vessels, called capillaries. The vital exchange of O_2 and CO_2 occurs by movement of these gases across the walls of the alveoli and small blood vessels.

Taking a Breath

With each breath, a bulk amount of air moves from outside the body through the nose and mouth into the windpipe, bronchial tubes, and air sacs. As we've noted, this inhalation of air is called inspiration. The movement of air is accomplished by the contraction of breathing muscles, which include the diaphragm and the muscles between the ribs, called intercostal. The muscle contractions produce expansion of the chest and lungs. Air moves due to a difference in pressure between the atmosphere and the chest. With exhalation of air, or expiration, the opposite process drives gases out of the lungs. The reverse movement of the diaphragm and intercostal muscles reduces the size of the lungs. Air moves out of the lungs due to a reversal in the pressure difference between the lung and atmosphere. Expiration is also aided by the elastic nature of the lung, which recoils after expansion.

Normal breathing involves a to-and-fro movement of air in and out of the lungs, which is produced with a minimal amount of energy. When breathing disorders occur, there is increased work of breathing as the muscle activity is increased. This increased energy demand of the respiratory muscles may produce the sensation of shortness of breath.

More Than Gas Exchange

Although the lung's primary function is the exchange of oxygen and carbon dioxide, many other tasks are also performed. Despite the fact that the lungs are located within the chest, they interact constantly with our environment. With each breath, the lungs are exposed to a large number of materials, including viruses, bacteria, pollens, and dust, as well as chemical-containing fumes that may be toxic.

HOW ARE THESE MATERIALS HANDLED?

To defend the body against the assault of these materials, the lungs are equipped with at least three dozen distinct types of cells, each assigned

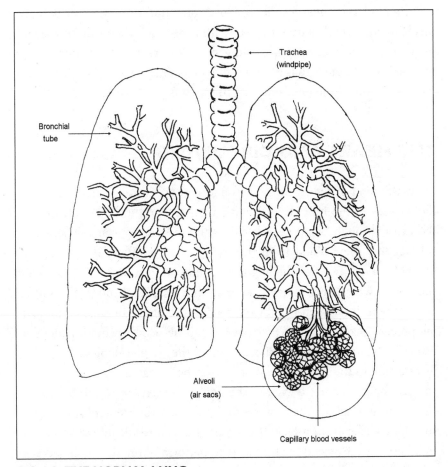

FIG. I.2 THE NORMAL LUNG.

to a special function. Some of these cells (macrophages) are scavengers that consume germs and foreign material. Many of the cells that line the bronchial tubes have delicate, hairlike projections, called cilia, which sweep back and forth, removing foreign invaders and material. Another type of lung cell produces sticky mucus, which traps germs and particles, allowing them to be removed by the expectoration of phlegm. Still other cells act on substances involved in the control of the body's blood pressure or as sentries to spot invading germs. The function of many other lung cells remains to be determined.

Many of the cells described above form the lung's natural defense mechanisms, which shield the body from disease. When these mechanisms are overwhelmed, breathing disorders result. Considering the number of pollutants that the lungs are constantly exposed to, it is striking that in most individuals normal function is preserved.

THE HEART AND CIRCULATION

Once the vital exchange of oxygen and carbon dioxide has occurred in the air sacs of the lung, the oxygen-enriched blood must be returned to the heart through blood vessels called the pulmonary veins. These vessels receive their blood from the many small capillary blood vessels. Once the blood reaches the heart, it is pumped into a large artery, called the aorta, which has major branches that extend through the entire body. When the oxygen-rich blood reaches the body's organs, an unloading process takes place so that the O_2 can be used as fuel for metabolism. The resulting carbon dioxide enters the oxygen-depleted blood to be returned to the lungs for the process to begin again.

The heart's action is vital to the delivery of oxygen to the body's tissues. Without an adequate pump to deliver fuel for metabolism, the tissues may suffer from a lack of oxygen, and as a result, organs may fail. In addition to the need for the heart to perform normally, the blood vessels of the circulation must be open to allow normal delivery. If there is obstruction of the arteries by plaque, which may form from cholesterol deposits, for example, the oxygen-rich blood may not reach the organs in adequate amounts.

RESPIRATORY FAILURE AND NORMAL LUNGS

The coordination of the brain centers, central and peripheral receptors, lung, and heart to produce the seemingly simple act of breathing is one of nature's remarkable feats. Although the most common causes of respiratory failure are diseases that attack the lungs themselves, failure may also occur in individuals with normal lungs. A tragic but increasingly frequent example is a drug overdose, whereby the brain centers cannot function and breathing ceases.

THE SPECTRUM OF LUNG DISEASE

An increasing number of disorders may disrupt the normal functioning of the lung, producing symptoms that often prompt medical evaluation. The causes of lung disease are diverse, ranging from air pollutants to carcinogens that trigger tumor growth and germs which produce infection. In many lung disorders, disease may be produced by an overreaction of the defending cells against an invader.

How Is Lung Disease Manifested?

A number of characteristic symptoms may signal the presence of a breathing disorder. In many instances, however, no symptoms may be manifested, and disease may be detected on a routine examination or chest x-ray. In some conditions, a high-pitched sound (wheeze) may be noted while exhaling. Cough may also be a striking and persistent symptom of chest disease. In some cases, a characteristic type of chest pain may be produced. The most frequently reported symptom of a breathing disorder, however, is shortness of breath.

AIR HUNGER

Because of the intricacy of the act of breathing, conflicting signals or increased demands may arise in a large number of disorders that affect the lungs, as well as the brain, heart, or respiratory muscles. These distress signals produce shortness of breath or air hunger. In some instances, shortness of breath may occur in the absence of lung disease. In Chapter 2, the meaning of shortness of breath will be explored.

2

SHORTNESS OF BREATH

WHAT DOES IT MEAN?

Shortness of breath is the subjective awareness of difficulty in breathing. Since breathing is normally automatic and effortless, this awareness is uncomfortable and unsettling. The medical term for shortness of breath is *dyspnea*, which is derived from the Greek meaning *bad breathing*. It is one of the most common symptoms for which patients seek medical attention.

Although shortness of breath is a sensation everyone has experienced, it should never be ignored because it may be an early signal of disease. In one large study of patients presenting to a lung clinic with shortness of breath, 75 percent were found to have a respiratory disorder. In more than half the patients with shortness of breath from lung disease, the cause was asthma or emphysema. Scarring of the lungs, called pulmonary fibrosis, was another major source of shortness of breath.

In the patients with shortness of breath who did not have lung disease, the causes included nasal congestion or rhinitis; heart disease; reflux of stomach acid; curvature of the spine, called kyphoscoliosis; and lack of physical conditioning. Anxiety was found to be the cause in 5 percent.

Edward G. was a thirty-two-year-old landscaper who first noted shortness of breath about one year before I saw him in consultation. Initially, the patient had noted breathing difficulty with exertion while working. He attributed the problem to overdoing it and not being in shape. Gradually, the problem progressed and Edward noted that he was breathless with routine activities, like showering or eating a heavy meal. At the time of consultation, he was unable to speak without breathlessness. Observing him during the interview, I noticed that he was breathing rapidly, taking small, shallow breaths. His physical examination and x-rays suggested pulmonary fibrosis, and the diagnosis was confirmed by lung biopsy. A trial of medical therapy that consisted of corticosteroids and other drugs which suppress the immune system failed. This therapy might have been effective if it had been initiated during the early stages of his disease. A lung transplant was recommended, but Edward died of pneumonia while waiting for a donor.

HOW IS SHORTNESS OF BREATH PRODUCED?

Distress Signals from the Bronchial Tubes

The most common causes of shortness of breath are diseases of the lung. As noted in Chapter 1, there are nerve receptors located in both the bronchial tubes, as well as in the walls of the alveoli. When the bronchial tubes are irritated, the bronchial receptors will fire and send a distress signal to the brain. This might occur in bronchial asthma, where there is inflammation in the air passages. The signals from the bronchial receptors are transmitted to neurons in the brain stem, which respond by increasing the rate of breathing. These and other neurons may also increase the size or depth of breathing or produce a cough or a sigh. The increase in rate and depth of breathing produces increased awareness of difficulty in breathing or shortness of breath.

Distress Signals from the Alveoli

Shortness of breath may also be produced by the firing of receptors located within the walls of the air sacs. One common example of the action of these receptors is when the alveoli fill with fluid. This might occur from weakening of the heart muscle, called congestive heart failure. Fluid is forced from the small blood vessels in the lung into the air sacs when the heart fails to pump the blood forward into the aorta and pressure is exerted backward into the vessels of the lung. Fluid in the lung is called pulmonary edema, and the presence of the fluid stimulates the lung receptors to fire. Once the distress signal is received by the brain, the breathing pattern is altered to produce rapid and shallow breaths. When this occurs, there is increased awareness of breathing or shortness of breath.

Signals from Outside the Lung

Lung diseases may also produce shortness of breath through other nerve pathways that do not originate in the lung. If a disease of the lung reduces oxygen or increases carbon dioxide, nerve signals will be sent from the carotid body and brain stem. These signals will also result in alterations in breathing and shortness of breath. Another pathway for the production of shortness of breath from receptors outside the lung exists in nerve connections from the muscles of breathing, such as the diaphragm. These receptors might fire if the position of the diaphragm is altered. This might occur after chest or abdominal surgery, resulting in this disturbing symptom.

Breathlessness without Lung Disease

Shortness of breath may also occur in the absence of lung disease. In a number of medical conditions, we see an increased sensitivity to oxygen and carbon dioxide levels producing shortness of breath. In these conditions, the rate and depth of breathing is increased during rest and exertion. One common example would be the presence of a high fever. Other examples include pregnancy, overactivity of the thyroid gland (hyperthyroidism), and overdosage of aspirin (salicylism).

IF THE NOSE CLOSES

A number of common conditions produce shortness of breath by blocking the nasal passages. In normal breathing, air enters through the nose. If the nostrils are closed, there is an almost immediate production of the sensation of shortness of breath by a nerve-reflex mechanism. Discomfort is also partly due to the necessity to breathe through the mouth.

A LACK OF FITNESS

Another common source of shortness of breath is a lack of fitness (conditioning), which is also described as being out of shape. A lack of regular exercise will often produce deconditioning and breathing distress with exertion. During exertion, greater demands are placed on the heart and lungs. Oxygen is the fuel required for muscles to function, and a greater amount is required during increased activity.

The human heart is a muscle that can be made stronger through regular exercise. As the heart muscle strengthens, it pumps more blood with each beat, providing greater amounts of oxygen to be used by the muscles as fuel. Fitness is often manifested by the development of a slower pulse rate because each pulsation of the heart is able to deliver more oxygen to the body's tissues. Many people sense conditioning as better stamina or less shortness of breath with exercise.

IS IT ANXIETY?

Anxiety is an emotional and physical response to a recognized threat. It is indistinguishable from fear. The intensity of anxiety varies greatly from minor qualms and noticeable trembling to even complete panic, the most extreme form.

An increased awareness of breathing is a common feature of anxiety. Patients with anxiety frequently present to physicians with the complaint of shortness of breath. In the severe form of anxiety, known as panic disorder, there may be hyperventilation. Patients may be unaware of the manifestations of their anxiety state and seek an examination to determine the physical nature of their complaint. Other patients may recognize anxiety but feel that their breathing disorder is unrelated.

Ten years ago I was asked to see a young woman in emergency consultation. She had noted severe shortness of breath for approximately one week. In addition to shortness of breath, she noted a "lump in my throat" and the sensation of being unable to swallow. At times, she was light-headed and had nearly fainted. The patient had already been seen by her internist, who had performed several routine tests, including a chest x-ray. She had undergone examinations of her throat and esophagus. All her tests had proved normal.

During the interview, I noted that the patient's breathing pattern was irregular. There were frequent deep breaths and sighs, and when I asked about them, she said, "I can't seem to get a full breath." During our conversation, the patient volunteered that she had been under tremendous pressure due to her recent marriage and a change in lifestyle. I ordered pulmonary function tests and a scan of her lungs. Both of the tests were normal and I referred the patient to a psychiatrist who concurred with a diagnosis of an acute anxiety disorder. After psychiatric intervention, the patient improved dramatically. I spoke to her a few weeks later, and she thanked me for directing her to therapy. In the course of our conversation she said, "I had no idea that stress could make my breathing so uncomfortable."

Although anxiety may produce the sensation of shortness of breath, more than 90 percent of patients with this complaint have a physical cause. Any patient with this complaint must have a thorough evaluation, as detailed in Chapter 3. Shortness of breath may be the only symptom of serious lung or heart disease and should never be ignored or attributed to anxiety without careful evaluation. The most common causes of shortness of breath are illustrated in Fig. 2.1.

A twenty-two-year-old woman consulted me four years ago for a complaint of shortness of breath. Shortly after our introductions, she said, "You're going to tell me I'm crazy." She added that she had been short-winded for several years and had seen several physicians, with normal results. The patient was unable to exercise and had restricted her lifestyle considerably. She noted a number of additional and varied

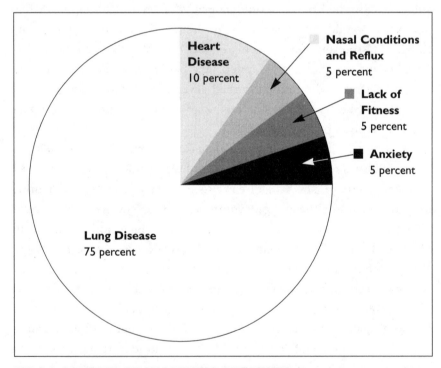

FIG. 2.1 SOURCES OF SHORTNESS OF BREATH.

complaints, including irritable bowel syndrome, and was under the care of a colon specialist. She was clearly nervous and ill at ease during the interview. She had also seen a heart specialist for palpitations.

It was easy to see why other physicians might have thought that her problems were all anxiety related. The patient mentioned that she often had a nasal drip, which made me suspect that she might be asthmatic. I inquired about allergies, but she was unaware of any and said that no one in her family had allergy or asthma. The patient's lung examination, x-ray, and electrocardiogram were all normal. Examination of her nose, however, revealed congestion and a small nasal polyp. I ordered pulmonary function tests, which confirmed that the patient was asthmatic. When I informed her of the diagnosis, she responded, "I knew I wasn't crazy." Now on a proper medical regimen, she has resumed exercise and is rarely short of breath.

THE NEXT STEP

To properly evaluate a patient with the complaint of shortness of breath, the physician must perform a detailed interview, physical, and laboratory examination. All the body's systems must be reviewed in order to avoid overlooking a non-respiratory cause of shortness of breath. Proceeding in this systematic manner can preclude misdiagnosis.

THE MEDICAL EVALUATION

Shortness of breath may signal the development of a breathing disorder and should never be ignored. Unfortunately, many patients may delay medical evaluation, and by doing so delay the diagnosis and treatment of a serious medical condition. Once the patient presents to the physician, a detailed evaluation should be performed to determine the nature of the problem.

The Medical Interview

The medical evaluation begins with taking a detailed medical history. From this history emerge vital details that point the physician toward formulating a diagnosis. Although the medical history focuses on the respiratory system, it is important that it be complete and comprehensive because the source of shortness of breath may not be pulmonary.

Although the interview is primarily conducted for recording the medical history, it is also part of the physical examination. A good observer may be able to make a diagnosis before even reaching the examination room. The nature and severity of shortness of breath may be evident in the patient's speech and body language. It may be difficult for patients with severe breathing disorders to speak without having to stop and rest. If oxygen levels are low, there may be a bluish discoloration of the lips, which is known as cyanosis. The patient's breathing pattern may also be evident during the examination. A fast but regular breathing pattern may signal lung or heart disease. The frequent clearing of the throat may be a sign of a postnasal drip. Irregular breathing with frequent sighs may be an indication of anxiety. Anxiety is normally present to a certain degree in any initial encounter in a physician's office, however, so the physician must observe if it is sustained throughout the interview.

THE IMPORTANT QUESTIONS

What It Feels Like

When a patient presents with a complaint of shortness of breath, the physician will ask specific questions to elucidate the nature of the problem. The first calls for the patient to describe the sensation: "What is it like?" Since shortness of breath is a subjective sensation, it will be described in many ways. One of the most common descriptions is a "suffocating" feeling or an inability to "catch my breath." Patients may describe a sensation of "not getting a full breath" and must sigh to achieve comfort. This sensation is best described as air hunger. The sensation of shortness of breath may be accompanied by chest discomfort (heaviness) and fatigue. Frequently, patients describe an anxiety reaction due to severe shortness of breath.

When and How It Started

After establishing the nature of the sensation, it is important to determine how long the problem has existed ("when did it start?") and whether it was sudden or gradual ("how did it start?"). Breathing disorders that have been present for a prolonged period, such as emphysema or fibrosis of the lung, are often described as beginning gradually over a period of several years. Patients with asthma, however, may experience the sudden onset of shortness of breath with an asthmatic attack.

What Makes It Happen?

One of the most important questions discerns whether the sensation is present continuously ("when does it occur?"). Shortness of breath is often only experienced with exertion, which increases the demands on the heart and lungs to supply adequate amounts of oxygen. It is important to try to quantify how much exertion is required to produce the symptom of shortness of breath. The physician may ask, "How many blocks can you walk before you have to stop?" or "How many flights of stairs can you climb without stopping?" The form of breathlessness that occurs only with exertion usually indicates a mild or early disorder.

Shortness of breath that is present at rest, however, always indicates a serious breathing disorder. This severe form of breathing difficulty is often the presenting symptom of patients with severe lung or heart disease. These patients experience a continuous struggle to breathe, which may interfere with simple daily activities, such as dressing, eating, and bathing. Many patients will describe having to stop several times while making their beds or taking a shower, for instance.

Is It Positional (Orthopnea)?

Another important question is whether shortness of breath occurs in different positions ("what happens when you lie down?" or "do you feel better in any particular position?"). Shortness of breath that occurs immediately upon assuming the recumbent position is called orthopnea. This striking feature is often described by patients as "I'm all right until I lie down." Orthopnea is often a characteristic of shortness of breath due to heart failure but may also occur in patients with lung disease or post-nasal drip. In patients with heart failure, this symptom occurs due to the return of blood from the lower limbs. The weakened heart is unable to pump the increased amount of returned blood, and fluid backs up into the lungs to produce shortness of breath. In patients with heart disease, this symptom always indicates a severe malfunction of the heart.

In some patients with heart disease, shortness of breath is not experienced immediately on assuming a recumbent position but occurs hours later. These patients are often awakened from a sound sleep with severe breathlessness that causes them to sit upright. Many patients describe opening a window to "get more air." This symptom is called paroxysmal nocturnal dyspnea, and it is characteristic of heart disease. The mechanism is similar to orthopnea, but in these patients the overload of fluid returning from the legs produces lung congestion more slowly.

Exploring Other Areas

The detailed history will also include important questions concerning childhood illnesses, allergy, sleep habits, smoking, and infections, and will review each of the body's many organ systems. The review of the heart and circulation will determine if the patient has a high risk of heart disease due to high blood pressure, smoking, diabetes, and high cholesterol. The physician will inquire as to whether illnesses such as asthma have occurred in the family, since a genetic predisposition has been established for this and other breathing disorders. A detailed occupational history is also important because the inhalation of materials such as coal dust and silica has been shown to produce scarring of the lungs. It is important to inquire about the patient's lifestyle. Patients who are very sedentary may experience shortness of breath because of a lack of conditioning.

The Physical Examination

After the medical history is taken, the physician proceeds to a detailed physical examination. As noted above, the exam really began during the interview, but the physician now has the opportunity to examine the patient more carefully. All organ systems are examined, but it is necessary to focus on certain areas in the evaluation of shortness of breath. Exams begin with the taking of the vital signs: blood pressure, heart rate (pulse), and the number of breaths per minute. Patients with severe problems will often have a fast pulse and rapid breathing. These patients may present a blue discoloration of the lips or nails (cyanosis). The nails may also reveal a characteristic curvature, called clubbing. This sign may indicate a low oxygen level but may also be hereditary or related to heart disease. The throat and nasal passages must be examined to determine that air may pass through easily. The finding of rhinitis or a deviated nasal septum, for example, may be important. The heart and lungs are examined carefully, looking for indications of disease. In some patients with shortness of breath, the examination may be entirely normal. In these patients, the problem may be mild or stem from anxiety.

X-Ray and Laboratory Evaluation

BLOOD TESTS

The laboratory evaluation of shortness of breath includes many of the routine lab tests, including blood count, blood chemistry, and urinalysis. One of the most common sources of shortness of breath is anemia. Here, the number of red blood cells and the hemoglobin they carry is reduced. Oxygen attaches to hemoglobin when it enters the small capillary blood vessel in the wall of the lung's air sacs. If there is not enough hemoglobin to carry the oxygen that has been inspired, the body tissues do not receive their required fuel. This occurs despite the normal functioning of the heart and lungs.

The routine blood count (CBC) may also signal the presence of a severe heart or lung problem. The human body can compensate for many abnormalities. One of these compensatory mechanisms is the response to a prolonged lack of oxygen. When oxygen levels are low, the body produces more red blood cells and hemoglobin. This is a slow process that requires days to weeks. This is the opposite of anemia and represents an attempt to increase the delivery of oxygen to the tissues.

Blood chemistry may signal a compensatory mechanism for elevated carbon dioxide levels. When CO_2 levels rise as a result of breathing disorders, there is a disturbance of the normal chemical balance of the blood. To buffer or balance this increase, a substance called bicarbonate is produced. The finding of an elevated bicarbonate level in the blood alerts the physician to the possibility of an increase in CO_2. Routine blood chemistry will also include blood sugar, cholesterol, liver, and kidney function. Abnormalities in these chemistries may point the physician toward a diagnostic abnormality. Elevations in liver tests, for example, in a patient presenting with shortness of breath may suggest the possibility of a disease known as sarcoidosis. (See Chapter 5.)

The physician may order many additional laboratory tests based on the patient's history and physical examination. The patient who has complained of breathlessness and who has a history of hay fever and corresponding physical findings will likely undergo allergy testing. This might consist of blood analysis or skin testing. If there is suspicion of a specific illness—such as sarcoidosis—additional blood tests will be performed.

THE CHEST X-RAY

In this high-tech era, one of the most helpful tools in the evaluation of shortness of breath is the chest x-ray. It is most useful in diseases of the lung, such as lung cancer, pulmonary fibrosis, emphysema, and infections, including pneumonia. The chest x-ray also provides vital information in patients with heart disease. A change in the heart's size or shape may indicate a cardiac problem. Clear indications of increased fluid in the blood vessels and air sacs of the lung may be seen in patients with heart failure.

A chest x-ray may also be helpful by being entirely normal. (See Fig. 2.2.) This may occur in patients with bronchial asthma, for example, whereby the abnormality producing breathlessness is located in the air passages, or bronchial tubes. These tubes are not easily seen on the chest x-ray. Another example in which the chest x-ray might be normal

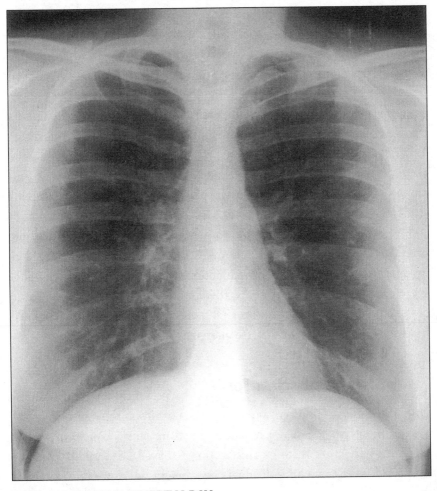

FIG. 2.2 A NORMAL CHEST X-RAY.

is in a patient who has experienced a blood clot or embolus in the lung. (See Chapter 6.)

CAT SCANNING

The physician may order additional and more detailed x-ray studies based on the initial examination. One example would be in evaluating the patient with shortness of breath and postnasal drip where a detailed x-ray of the nasal and sinus passages is needed. A computer-programmed study, called a CAT scan, might reveal a deviated nasal septum or blockage of the passages by fleshy growths, called polyps. CAT scanning of the lungs might also be helpful in detecting early stages of diseases such as emphysema, pulmonary fibrosis, and lung cancer. A chest CAT scan is a series of three-dimensional x-ray images obtained with the patient lying on an x-ray table. The scanner is programmed to obtain images from the neck, down to the abdomen. The scanned images are taken at a distance of only a few millimeters apart. The closer the images, the more detailed the scan. In the evaluation of lung disorders, such as pulmonary fibrosis, it is common for the physician to order a "thin section" study in which the images are very close together.

A CAT scan may be done with or without the injection of a contrast dye. This material is injected into a vein in the patient's arm, and the x-ray images are obtained as the dye courses through the blood vessels of the chest. In some lung diseases, this contrast agent may be helpful in obtaining an accurate diagnosis. This method will not be used routinely, however, since the dye may cause allergic reactions.

Pulmonary Function Tests

One of the most important methods of determining the cause of shortness of breath is a series of breathing measurements, commonly called pulmonary function testing. This testing is based on normal standards that are derived from an individual's age, height, weight, and sex. These values enable physicians to predict the patient's breathing capacity. The results are often expressed as a percentage of what has been predicted. A complete study of lung function usually includes spirometry, lung volumes, and a diffusion capacity.

SPIROMETRY

One of the simplest yet most revealing tests of lung function is spirometry. Here, a patient is asked to inhale deeply and to exhale forcefully for as long as possible. The amount of air exhaled by this maximum effort is called the vital capacity. Vital capacity may be affected by many forms of breathing disorders. Spirometry also measures how quickly the air is expelled and compares the "airflow" to normal standards. A commonly used airflow measurement is the maximum, or peak flow, that can be generated. Reductions in airflow may reflect a narrowing of the bronchial tubes. Narrowing of the air passages may occur in emphysema, bronchitis, and bronchial asthma. To determine if this narrowing is due to the constriction seen in bronchial asthma, spirometry is performed before and after the inhalation of a bronchodilator medication. In the asthmatic, this medication will significantly open or dilate the bronchial tubes. A significant response to bronchodilator medication is defined as at least a 15 percent improvement in airflows.

LUNG VOLUMES

Spirometry may reveal abnormalities in vital capacity and airflows that do not indicate a specific diagnosis. In these patients, further information is needed to determine the source of shortness of breath. Another useful test is the measurement of how air is distributed in the lung. This is called lung volumes.

In the normal lung, air is distributed in several divisions, or compartments. One example is the amount of air that is exchanged with each breath, called the tidal volume. Another important lung compartment is the constant amount of air that remains in the air sacs at all times. This division is called the residual volume. If the physician can detect a change in the distribution of air, a pattern of disease may emerge, which leads to a specific diagnosis. In emphysema, for example, air is often "trapped" in large air sacs, producing an increase in residual volume.

Lung volumes may be measured by two methods. A commonly used technique requires the patient to breathe for several minutes a special gas mixture containing helium. Lung volumes can then be calculated from the amount of helium exhaled. Another method requires the use of a glass booth, called a plethysmograph. In this method, the patient sits in the "body box" and breathes against a mouthpiece. By analyzing pressure changes in the box as the patient breathes, it is possible to determine the volume of gas in the lungs.

DIFFUSION CAPACITY

Another important test of lung function is called the diffusion capacity. Here, the physician determines how well gas is exchanged or transferred from the lung's air sacs to the blood vessels. This requires the patient to breathe a special gas mixture containing carbon monoxide (CO) and the exhaled air is analyzed. The difference in CO in the inhaled and exhaled air is the amount that transferred into the blood. The diffusion capacity is a sensitive test for breathing disorders—such as emphysema and pulmonary fibrosis—that affect the air sacs, or alveoli.

EXERCISE TESTING

Spirometry, lung volumes, and diffusion capacity are all performed at rest. In many patients, shortness of breath may only be experienced on exertion. An exercise test may help determine the source of shortness of breath in these patients. One example is the asthmatic patient who experiences constriction of the bronchial tubes only with exertion (exercise-induced asthma). In these patients, spirometry performed after exercise reveals a significant reduction in airflows.

Exercise testing is performed with either a stationary bicycle or a treadmill. The patient is asked to slowly increase the level of exercise until a certain heart rate is achieved or shortness of breath develops. During the test, the physician normally monitors blood pressure, oxygen levels, breathing rate, and the electrocardiogram (EKG), which is a tracing of the heart's electrical activity.

Exercise produces an increase in the amount of oxygen taken up by the body's muscles. The maximum amount of oxygen that is used is called the maximum oxygen uptake (VO_2). This measurement is the standard for determining fitness. The greater the value, the better conditioned the individual. Normal standards for the amount of exercise, oxygen uptake, heart rate, and breathing function are used in the evaluation of an exercise test. By comparing the patient's performance with the normal standards, it is possible to determine if the source of breathlessness is related to heart or lung disease or to a lack of conditioning.

Exercise testing may also be used specifically to assess heart performance. Examples of how exercise testing may be used in determining the function of the heart are offered below.

Arterial Blood Gases and Oximetry

One of the most helpful measurements of lung function is the direct determination of the levels of oxygen and carbon dioxide in the blood, which is known as a blood gas. Slight changes in these levels may be an early indication of a breathing disorder. The absolute levels of oxygen and carbon dioxide may often indicate the severity of the breathing disorder and its prognosis. In patients with severe abnormalities in O_2 and CO_2 levels, a mechanical respirator may be necessary.

To measure these levels, it is necessary to obtain blood from an artery. Arterial blood is the enriched blood that has been returned to the heart from the lungs after gas exchange and then pumped by the heart into the body's circulation. It is common practice to obtain the arterial blood gas from the radial artery, which is located at the wrist.

Blood oxygen levels may also be measured by a less invasive technique known as oximetry. This bloodless method requires a sensor called an oximeter to be placed over a fingernail or on the earlobe. The oximeter transmits different wavelengths of light through the small blood vessels, called capillaries. In the fingernail and earlobe, these blood vessels are close to the surface of the skin. In these small vessels, oxygen is carried by a protein, called hemoglobin. As the body uses oxygen, the hemoglobin undergoes a change that an oximeter detects as a different absorption of light. This determination, called oxygen saturation, is made during each pulse beat and from the relative amounts of hemoglobin with and without oxygen. Oximetry does not measure carbon dioxide levels, so a blood gas may still be necessary in some patients.

Lung Biopsy

In many patients, the diagnosis of a breathing disorder may require an actual sampling of the lung tissue; this is called a lung biopsy. In these patients, the chest x-ray or CAT scan, as well as laboratory and breathing function tests, do not determine the specific lung disorder. Although this is a more invasive approach, the accuracy of diagnosis provided by lung biopsy is high and the information gained by this approach may be invaluable.

Lung biopsies may be obtained by several methods. Two commonly used techniques are bronchoscopy and needle biopsy. Both may be performed in the outpatient setting in suitable patients.

BRONCHOSCOPY

Bronchoscopy, a technique for the examination of the bronchial tubes, was originally performed with hollow, stiff metal instruments. In the last eighteen years, this technique has been radically changed by the development of flexible fiberoptic instruments. This fiberscope is a narrow tube with a diameter of approximately 6 millimeters and can be easily passed deep into the many branches of the bronchial tubes. It has an inner channel that is used for inserting and moving wire instruments, as well as for suctioning secretions. The wire instruments can be manipulated to obtain samples of the bronchial tubes, as well as of the air sacs. Using a guiding x-ray, called a fluoroscope, the physician can direct the bronchoscope to the area of lung that requires sampling.

NEEDLE BIOPSY

In selected patients, an alternative technique called a needle biopsy may be preferred. Under local anesthesia, a thin needle is inserted through the skin into the lung and a sample is aspirated into a syringe. Needle biopsy is commonly done with the guidance of a CAT scan image, which can direct the physician to the most accurate placement of the needle.

Needle biopsy is most helpful in the diagnosis of lung cancer, especially when the tumor is located close to the outer portion of the lung. In these patients, the bronchoscope may not be able to reach and sample the involved area as accurately.

Both bronchoscopic and needle biopsy of the lung are limited by the small sample size that is obtained. In many lung diseases, a small sample is inadequate for an accurate diagnosis. In patients with these diseases, a larger sample must be obtained surgically.

OPEN-LUNG BIOPSY

In order to obtain a larger sample of the lung for diagnosis, an incision must be made in the chest. This technique is often called an open-lung biopsy. In the last several years, a less invasive surgical technique, known as thoracoscopy, has been used. In thoracoscopy, the physician makes a small opening between two ribs and inserts a metal scope through which the lung sample is withdrawn. To provide direction, a video probe may also be inserted into the chest through another opening. Although this technique is less surgically invasive, it still requires general anesthesia and is performed in an operating room.

Tests of Heart Performance

In the evaluation of shortness of breath, it may be necessary to perform tests of heart performance to determine if the source of the problem is heart disease. Many noninvasive tests are available to the physician.

ECHOCARDIOGRAPHY

One commonly used test is an echocardiogram, whereby sound waves are used to produce an image of the heart and its chambers. This test is performed by placing a sound probe in various positions on the front of the chest. This technique can determine how well the heart muscle contracts as it ejects blood into the circulation. Unfortunately, echocardiography does not obtain high-quality images in as many as 5 percent of patients tested, especially those with emphysema, deformities of the chest wall, and obesity. In these patients, sound may not penetrate adequately to produce the needed images. A new technique, called transesophageal echocardiography (TEE), in which the patient swallows a small sound probe, has made the examination of these patients more reliable.

NUCLEAR TESTS

When an echocardiogram does not provide accurate information on the performance of the heart, a nuclear imaging test may be performed.

Nuclear imaging tests involve the injection of small amounts of a radioactive substance and the use of a camera that can record radioactivity. By following the radioactive substance in the blood as it passes through the heart, the amount of blood ejected by the heart muscle can be calculated. This amount is compared with normal standards, and an assessment of the function of the heart is offered.

CARDIAC STRESS TESTING

An exercise test specifically designed to determine heart function may be required in the evaluation of shortness of breath. In many patients with heart disease, breathlessness is only noted with exertion. This exercise or stress test is usually performed with a treadmill with specialized monitoring of the heart. The most simple but useful form of monitoring is the use of the electrocardiogram.

Stress testing is often used in the evaluation of the patient suspected of having coronary artery disease. The coronary arteries are the blood vessels that supply oxygen to the heart. If these arteries become narrowed by fat deposits, called plaque, blood supply to the heart muscle decreases. When, during exercise, the demands of the heart muscle increase, the narrowed arteries may not be capable of supplying adequate oxygen. This lack of oxygen will produce significant changes on the electrocardiogram, which alert the physician to a lack of blood supply to the heart muscle.

Echocardiography and nuclear imaging may be combined with exercise testing to provide more detailed information about heart performance. In this combined test, an echocardiogram or nuclear image is obtained when the patient reaches the maximum exercise level.

CARDIAC CATHETERIZATION

A more invasive test of heart function may occasionally be required in the evaluation of a patient with shortness of breath. In cardiac catheterization, a thin plastic catheter is inserted into a blood vessel in the groin and advanced into the heart and great blood vessels.

It is helpful to think of the heart as having a left and right side. The right side of the heart receives the oxygen-depleted blood that is returning from the limbs and organs. This blood is then pumped into a large vessel, called the pulmonary artery. The pulmonary artery divides to serve both the right and left lung. The smallest branches of the pulmonary artery are the tiny capillary vessels that course between the alveoli to exchange oxygen and carbon dioxide. The oxygen-enriched blood then enters larger vessels, called pulmonary veins, which return blood to the left side of the heart. This returned blood is then pumped into the major artery, called the aorta, which divides to supply the entire circulation.

The catheter that is passed during catheterization is used to measure pressures within the heart's chambers, as well as the blood vessels entering and leaving the heart. These pressures may be useful in determining the function of the heart. By measuring the pressure within the pulmonary artery, the physician may also be able to assess the state of the many vessels that comprise the circulation within the lungs.

During catheterization, a dye may be injected to outline the coronary blood vessels. This procedure, called coronary angiography, is the most accurate method of determining whether these vessels are narrowed or blocked. If the physician suspects that the patient's shortness of breath is due to blood clots or emboli, dye may also be injected into the pulmonary artery and its branches. This procedure is known as a pulmonary angiogram.

AFTER THE MEDICAL EVALUATION: A DIAGNOSIS

The physician analyzes the results of this comprehensive medical evaluation of the patient with shortness of breath to arrive at a firm diagnosis. In many patients, this is accomplished in the examination room or after preliminary test results are reviewed. In some patients, however, further testing—such as pulmonary function tests, blood gases, exercise testing, lung biopsy, and tests of heart performance—is necessary to establish the cause of air hunger.

In the next chapters, specific disorders that produce breathlessness will be discussed.

3

DISEASES OF THE AIR PASSAGES

The respiratory tract is a passageway that extends from the nose or mouth to the lung's air sacs. Shortness of breath may occur when any portion of this tract is affected by disease. The voice box, or larynx, divides the respiratory tract into two portions, the upper and lower. This chapter will discuss the most common disorders that affect these vital air passages.

THE UPPER RESPIRATORY TRACT

The upper respiratory tract lies between the opening of the nose or mouth and the voice box. This area begins with either the two nasal cavities or the mouth and extends into the back of the throat, called the pharynx, which leads to the larynx. (See Fig. 3.1.) The nasal passages have openings called meati, which connect with the sinuses, cavelike structures in the skull located above and below the eyes. The sinuses serve many functions, including maintaining a constant temperature in the nasal passages.

The lining, called the mucosa, of the upper respiratory tract is a thin membrane that continues into the lower tract. This delicate membrane is composed of cells that are capable of secreting mucus. Small blood vessels are also distributed in the lining of the upper respiratory tract.

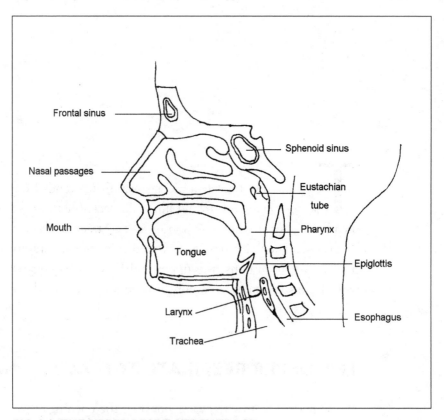

FIG. 3.1 THE UPPER RESPIRATORY TRACT.

These vessels are uniquely designed to warm the air that enters this passageway and are richly supplied with nerve endings. These nervous system connections provide the upper respiratory tract's ability to adapt rapidly to changes in the air that is inhaled.

The upper respiratory tract plays an important role in the act of breathing by regulating the size of the air passages. With inspiration, the passageways increase in size, allowing more air to enter the lungs. The reverse occurs in expiration. These changes are accomplished through the action of muscles located in the upper respiratory tract, as well as the diaphragm.

Why Breathe through the Nose?

Although the nose is significantly narrower than the mouth, nasal breathing is preferred. The nose is both an air conditioner and an important filter that serves to trap particles which are inhaled. These particles may be infectious organisms or a variety of air pollutants that would prove harmful if inhaled. The nose is also capable of absorbing potentially harmful gases, such as sulfur dioxide.

The nasal passage may change in size in response to a variety of stimuli. For example, exposure to cold air produces an almost instantaneous increase in blood in the nasal vessels. The passageway of the nose is also altered by a change in position. In the recumbent position, the nasal passage is narrower. With exercise, the nasal passage widens to allow more air to enter. With high levels of exercise, however, there is a reflex switch to mouth breathing.

Reflex closure of the nasal passages may also occur. When blowing out a candle, for example, a fleshy portion of the roof of the mouth, called the soft palate, may effectively close off the nasal passages. A natural narrowing of alternating sides of the nose occurs every three to four hours, so that one side appears to open while the other closes. This is a normal pattern, which many individuals interpret as illness. ("One side of my nose is always closed.") The cause of this change is unknown.

RHINITIS

Rhinitis may be defined as an inflammation of the lining of the nasal passages. It is a common occurrence, affecting an estimated 20 percent of the population.

Although not a life-threatening condition, rhinitis often produces severe symptoms of stuffiness, drip, sneezing, and itching. A severe episode may, in fact, be incapacitating. When nasal congestion is severe and the nasal passages are narrowed or obstructed, the patient may also complain of shortness of breath.

Determining the Cause

Rhinitis may be caused by a number of conditions. (See Table 3.1.) The physician is charged with the task of determining the cause in order to specify treatment. In the medical interview, the physician inquires about seasons in which the patient's symptoms may occur. Many patients with allergy to pollens have specific months of the year when they are symptomatic. In the Northeast, for example, the hay fever season, when ragweed pollen counts are highest, extends from mid-August to the first frost. In some patients, symptoms may occur every day of the year, regardless of the season. This form of rhinitis is called perennial, and it may be allergic or nonallergic.

The physician will also inquire as to whether the patient has a history of allergy or has ever reacted to animal dander, dust, pollens, medicines, or foods. Recent research has identified an allergy gene. The physician will inquire as to whether family members have had allergy, rhinitis, or asthma.

The physical examination of the nasal passages is the next step. This examination requires the physician to examine the nasal lining. The outer portion of the nose may be easily inspected with a light source. This is often aided by the use of an instrument called a speculum, which widens the nasal passageway. A helpful tool for the examination

---

TABLE 3.1 COMMON CAUSES OF RHINITIS

---

1. ALLERGIC
   a. Seasonal: pollens
   b. Perennial: dust mite, cockroach, animal dander, mold

2. NONALLERGIC
   a. Perennial: nasal polyps, irritants (cigarette smoke, fumes), infections, aging, sarcoidosis, cold air

3. RHINITIS MEDICAMENTOSA
   a. Decongestant nasal sprays
   b. Cocaine
   c. Beta-blocker medication (used for blood pressure, heart disease)
   d. Oral contraceptives

4. MISCELLANEOUS
   a. Reflex: change in position, bright lights, eating, sexual arousal
   b. Hormonal: underactive thyroid (hypothyroidism), pregnancy

---

of the back of the nose and the rest of the upper respiratory tract is a fiberoptic instrument, called the rhinoscope. This instrument resembles the bronchoscope but is much smaller. It can be passed easily into the nasal passages, requiring only a topical anesthetic.

After the physical examination, the physician will order appropriate laboratory tests. These might include skin testing or blood assay to test for allergy.

WHAT IS ALLERGY?

Allergy is a state of the body's hypersensitivity to a specific substance, called an allergen. Allergens may be inhaled, eaten, or injected. As noted, allergy has a genetic basis. In a susceptible individual, exposure to an allergen produces a chain reaction that results in a specific response. In some individuals, the response may be the symptoms of rhinitis.

Immunoglobulin E

The allergic reaction begins with the production of a blood protein substance, called Immunoglobulin E (IgE). This protein is specific for the exciting allergen. On exposure to the allergen, IgE attaches to the surface of allergy cells, called mast cells, causing their disintegration. When mast cells disintegrate, irritating chemicals are released and produce inflammation.

The total level of IgE in the blood may be measured. This is a useful screening test that the physician may use to identify an allergic individual. Unfortunately, this test may fail to identify some patients with allergy.

Levels of IgE for specific allergens may also be measured through blood testing. This technique is called RAST (Radioallergosorbent test) testing. RAST testing may be used to identify allergy to many allergens. In some patients, identification of allergy to a specific substance allows them to avoid or minimize exposure to the offending material.

Skin Testing

Although allergy skin testing has been used for more than a hundred years, it remains the most useful and cost-effective approach to allergy testing. Many considered it to be more reliable than blood testing. Skin testing is performed by pricking, scratching, or injecting the skin with a small amount of allergen. Positive reactions, which resemble hives, are noted in twenty to thirty minutes. Skin testing, however, is time consuming and may cause total-body reactions in highly sensitive individuals.

Nasal Smears

In the evaluation of rhinitis, the physician may obtain with a cotton-tipped swab a specimen of the nasal mucus and smear it on a glass slide. Under the microscope, this nasal smear may reveal the presence of allergy cells called eosinophils. The finding of increased numbers of these cells may confirm the diagnosis of allergic rhinitis.

Nasal Biopsy
In rare forms of rhinitis, a biopsy of the lining of the nasal passage is necessary for diagnosis. One such illness is sarcoidosis, which is discussed in the next chapter.

Allergic Rhinitis

Allergic rhinitis usually begins in childhood or adolescence but may occur at any time. It is often manifested as an immediate allergic reaction, such as a sneeze or exposure to inhaled allergens, including grass, ragweed, and tree pollens. Allergy to indoor allergens, such as animal dander, dust, dust mites, and molds, may produce year-round or perennial symptoms. Allergic rhinitis may also affect susceptible individuals, such as veterinarians or pharmaceutical workers.

The patient may complain of itching of the eyes, nose, roof of the mouth, and throat. This is less common in nonallergic rhinitis. Patients with severe stuffiness complain of breathlessness. A constant watery nasal drip is a frequent complaint. In children, this is often the source of an "allergy salute," as a hand is used to wipe the nose. On examination, the lining of the nasal passages appears swollen, with a clear watery discharge or drip. The patient's eyes are often red and infected.

TREATMENT OF ALLERGIC RHINITIS

The treatment of allergic rhinitis includes avoidance of offending allergens; medication; and desensitization, or immunotherapy, in selected individuals.

Avoidance
Although it is a simple and logical approach to allergic problems, avoidance is often not used to its full advantage in many patients. In patients with specific allergies, avoidance may lead to a marked reduction in symptoms. Table 3.2 lists some practical allergy-control measures.

Pollens and Molds

Pollens are seasonal, so patients should be able to prepare for particularly difficult months. Allergy testing may identify the specific pollens to be avoided. Pollen and mold-spore counts are usually available through news reports. Many organizations now offer this information through the Internet. (See the appendix.) Sensitive individuals are best protected by remaining indoors in an air-conditioned environment that contains an air filter.

Air filters may be mechanical or electrical. One of the best mechanical types incorporates a High Efficiency Particulate Air (HEPA) filter. These come in various sizes according to the volume of the room (amount of air) that must be filtered and circulated. Before you purchase one, know the dimensions of the room in which the air filter will be placed. One example of an electrical filter is the electrostatic precipitator. These filters and the HEPA filter can be placed in a home's central forced-air system. Electrical filters require more frequent cleaning than do mechanical filters.

Molds are fungi that grow well in warm and moist environments. They may be plentiful in the warmer months. Thousands of different species of mold exist. They may be found in high numbers on both dry and rainy days. *Alternaria* is a mold often found in dry, warm climates and in farming areas. *Fusarium* is a mold found on plants and is abundant during damp, humid weather. Other molds are found in decaying wood and soil. Anticipate exposure during outdoor activities (mowing the lawn, raking leaves). A simple face mask may help to reduce exposure. Sunglasses may also be helpful to reduce eye irritation due to pollens and molds.

Molds may also be found indoors, most commonly in the bathroom, kitchen, and basement. A useful step is to reduce humidity levels to 20 to 50 percent with a dehumidifier. The dehumidifier must be cleaned and emptied regularly. Since molds grow best in warm environments, an air conditioner may be helpful. Ventilation can help reduce mold-spore inhalation. An exhaust fan in the bathroom and kitchen may also reduce humidity levels.

Chemical sprays can kill mold and prevent its regrowth in highly susceptible areas (showers, basements, air conditioners, etc.). The appendix contains useful information for obtaining these materials.

Houseplants are not a major source of mold spores but are best kept to a minimum, since they increase humidity levels. Spores are often liberated when the plants are potted or watered.

Animal Allergens

Animal allergens are potent triggers of allergic rhinitis and are commonly found in homes or offices of pet owners because they can stick to clothing and be carried to any location outside of the home. The allergens consist of dander and saliva and are not related to breed or coat length. All breeds of cat, for example, share a common allergen, which may become airborne or be present in mattresses, carpets, bedcovers, and pillows.

The best way to reduce animal allergens is to get rid of the animal. Restricting a pet to a certain room or a portion of the home does not prevent airborne particles from spreading throughout the home. Even after the pet has been removed, allergens may remain for several months. An air filter may help to reduce airborne allergens. Cleaning with 3 percent tannic acid solution can denature residual animal allergen. Cat allergen has been demonstrated to remain for years at significant levels in mattresses. If you cannot part with your pet, a mattress and pillow cover are helpful for encasing animal allergens. Washing a cat weekly will reduce dander levels. This will be difficult at first, but cats can be gradually introduced to bathing by starting with one area at a time. The animal's coat can be treated with a spray or solution that reduces exposure to allergens. (See the appendix.)

Do not forget small pets—birds or rodents—which may also be the source of allergens that trigger allergic rhinitis.

Dust Mites

Dust mites are an important indoor trigger for allergic rhinitis. These tiny insects depend on moisture for survival and live on human skin dander. They have been found in abundant quantities in mattresses, pillows, clothes, bedcovers, carpets, towels, and even stuffed animals. In the home, the highest concentrations have been found in the bedroom. It is the feces of the dust mite that produces an allergic reaction. When dust is disturbed, these droppings become airborne and cause allergic reactions.

The particles are large enough to be trapped, however, and the patient can significantly reduce the number of dust mites through specific measures, including using a zippered mattress and pillow cover. Sheets and bedcovers should be washed weekly in hot water. Carpeting should be removed wherever possible, and remaining carpeting treated with a chemical agent, such as benzyl benzoate (Acarosan), or tannic acid, which kills mites. (See the appendix for more information on obtaining these materials.)

Vacuuming is important and should be done once a week, preferably not by the individual with allergic rhinitis. If you must vacuum yourself, use a dust mask and a vacuum cleaner with high-density paper bags and filtration, as well as a HEPA filter. Indoor humidity levels should be reduced to less than 50 percent with a dehumidifier; an air filter should be placed in the bedroom.

Medication for Allergic Rhinitis
Many useful medications are available for the treatment of allergic rhinitis. The physician should individualize a treatment program for each patient. As with all medication programs, a review of possible adverse effects must be performed.

■ Decongestants
In patients with mild allergic rhinitis, a decongestant or antihistamine alone or in combination may be sufficient. Decongestants, such as pseudoephedrine, work by constricting the swollen blood vessels in the nasal passages. The result is decreased congestion and a wider passageway. Whenever possible, decongestants should be taken by mouth because the prolonged application of a topical spray may result in increased congestion (see below). If a topical spray is needed, it should

---

TABLE 3.2 ALLERGY-CONTROL MEASURES

INDOOR ALLERGENS

Dust mites

- Encase bedding in airtight, dust-proof covers

- Wash bedding in water hotter than 130 degrees F.

- Remove wall-to-wall carpeting

- Use HEPA air filter

Mold

- Destroy moisture-prone areas

- Avoid high humidity in bedroom

- Check basement and attic for standing water and mold

Cockroaches

- Control available food supply

- Professionally exterminate

OUTDOOR ALLERGENS

Pollen

- Keep car and house windows closed

- Use air conditioning and HEPA air filter

- Time outdoor exposures and activities

---

not be used for more than four days. Adverse effects of decongestants include dryness of the mouth and mucous membranes, insomnia, nervousness, high blood pressure, headache, and palpitations. Their use may be contraindicated in patients with high blood pressure or heart disease and in selected patients with asthma. Many decongestants are available for sale over the counter, often in combination with antihistamines. Whenever possible, their use should be discussed with a physician.

Antihistamines

Histamine is an irritating chemical substance that is liberated from destroyed allergy cells. Antihistamines bind to histamine and neutralize its effects. These medications can be taken orally and in many patients are capable of effectively reducing symptoms. Many of the original antihistamine medications, such as Benadryl and ChlorTrimeton, are available without prescription. These medications produce drowsiness, which may limit their use. In the last eight years, a second generation of antihistamines has been developed; these medications are much less likely to produce sedation, and are also longer acting and usually administered once or twice a day. Examples include astemizole (Hismanal), cetirizine (Zyrtec), fexofenadine (Allegra), loratadine (Claritin), and terfenadine (Seldane). (Terfenadine has recently been withdrawn due to drug interactions and rare cases of irregular heart rhythm.) The adverse effects of antihistamines as a group include headache, somnolence, dry mouth, and altered urination. Their use may be contraindicated in selected patients with asthma and in patients with urinary problems, such as an enlarged prostate.

Cromolyn Sodium

Allergic rhinitis may not respond adequately to the use of decongestants and antihistamines. In these patients, the use of either cromolyn sodium (Nasalcrom) or a topical corticosteroid spray should be considered. Both of these agents reduce inflammation of the nasal mucosa. Cromolyn sodium is a unique chemical substance derived from khellin, an Egyptian herbal remedy. Its mechanism of action is unclear, but speculation has centered on the stabilizing effect of cromolyn on mast cells. Cromolyn is applied to the nose as a nasal spray three to four times daily. It is not immediately effective and may require two to four weeks to achieve its maximum effect. Because of this mode of action, cromolyn sodium is best started two to three weeks before the onset of the pollen season. Adverse effects include sneezing and a mild burning sensation with its application. Cromolyn sodium is approved for children six years of age and older.

Topical Corticosteroids

Topical corticosteroid sprays are widely used for patients with allergic rhinitis that is difficult to control. These agents reduce inflammation in the nasal passages by reducing the number of allergy cells. Although their onset of action is faster than cromolyn sodium, an effect is often not felt for three days and peaks after two to three weeks of use. Examples of the steroid sprays available in the United States are beclomethasone (Vancenase, Beconase), budesonide (Rhinocort), fluticasone (Flonase), flunisolide (Nasalide), mometasone (Nasonex), and triamcinolone (Nasacort). These agents are often administered once or twice a day. The most common adverse effect of the topical steroid sprays is a stinging sensation noted on application. Sneezing and nasal bleeding (epistaxis) have been infrequently noted.

The topical corticosteroid nasal sprays have not been shown to have any total-body side effects. Their action is local on the mucosa of the nasal passages, and little blood absorption has been found. Many of these medications were originally available as skin creams and lotions, and their safety is similar to the many steroid preparations that are applied to the skin.

Immunotherapy

Allergy treatment or immunotherapy may be helpful in selected patients with allergic rhinitis. It is indicated in the allergic individual who has failed medical therapy or who is unable to tolerate the above medications.

Immunotherapy, or desensitization, involves the injection of minute amounts of specific allergens. Allergy shots are only given after sensitivity to specific allergens has been identified. The amount of the allergen is slowly increased in the allergy injection so that a "blocking antibody" that can interrupt the allergic reaction may be produced. Studies of immunotherapy in patients with allergic rhinitis have shown a significant reduction in symptoms. This treatment is a gradual process, however, often requiring weeks to months to achieve a response. In older subjects, the response to treatment may not be as pronounced as in younger patients. In sensitive individuals, a generalized allergic reaction may develop after the administration of allergens, preventing the continuation of treatment.

WHY TREAT ALLERGIC RHINITIS?

For many individuals, allergic rhinitis is regarded as a nuisance rather than a disease. Many patients feel they can "live with it," since the disorder is not life threatening. One of the most convincing arguments for the treatment of allergic rhinitis, however, comes from research that has linked this condition to both sinusitis, inflammation in the sinus cavities, and asthma.

Studies have shown how allergic rhinitis can cause sinusitis. When the lining of the nose becomes swollen after exposure to allergens, the openings to the sinuses become narrowed or closed. The decreased air entry into the sinus cavities promotes the development of inflammation and sinus infection.

Allergic rhinitis may also be regarded as a risk factor for the development of bronchial asthma. In one study of allergic rhinitis, 10.5 percent of the patients developed asthma over a twenty-three-year period. More importantly, several studies of patients with both allergic rhinitis and bronchial asthma have shown that treatment of rhinitis improves the management of the patient's asthma.

These studies strongly support the vigorous treatment of allergic rhinitis.

Nonallergic Rhinitis

Nonallergic rhinitis has its onset later in life than the allergic type. Symptoms of nasal stuffiness, watery drip, sneezing, and shortness of breath may cause the patient to seek medical attention. Itching is uncommon in these patients. Symptoms usually occur throughout the year.

On physical examination, the nasal mucosa may reveal swelling and redness or appear normal. Serum IgE is normal and allergy tests are negative. These patients do not have a family history of allergy or rhinitis.

TREATMENT OF NONALLERGIC RHINITIS

The treatment of nonallergic rhinitis may include many of the agents listed for treatment of the allergic type. Many patients will respond to decongestants and antihistamines. A topical corticosteroid spray may also be effective.

Ipratropium Bromide

Ipratropium bromide (Atrovent) has proved useful in the treatment of nonallergic rhinitis. This medication is applied as a spray and works by interrupting nerve signals that control the amount of blood contained in the small blood vessels of the nasal lining. Adverse effects include headache, dryness of the mouth, and urinary difficulty. Ipratropium bromide is also used as a bronchodilator medication in patients with lower respiratory tract disease. (See below.)

Rhinitis Medicamentosa

Rhinitis medicamentosa is common and results from the use of a specific medication. This condition often presents severe nasal congestion and may produce shortness of breath.

One of the most severe examples of rhinitis medicamentosa results from the use of over-the-counter decongestant nasal sprays. These sprays contain potent agents called vasoconstrictors, which act on the many small blood vessels in the nasal passage. The vasoconstrictor reduces the amount of blood in these vessels, causing decreased swelling and congestion. Although initially beneficial, the continued application (used regularly for more than four days) of this type of medication often results in a "rebound" increase in blood flow to these blood vessels. The increased blood flow increases congestion, resulting in a reapplication of the offending medication.

Many patients with rhinitis medicamentosa report that they feel "trapped by the medication" since it is "the only thing that opens my nose." When informed that it is, in fact, the cause of the problem, most patients seek proper treatment.

TREATMENT OF RHINITIS MEDICAMENTOSA

Rhinitis medicamentosa can be prevented by limiting how long a decongestant nasal spray is used. Regular use should be limited to no more than four days. Once this condition is established, it is best treated by discontinuing the spray and administering an oral decongestant, such as pseudoephedrine. A topical corticosteroid spray is often also effective.

NASAL POLYPS

Nasal polyps are a frequent cause of obstruction of the nasal passages. They are pale, gelatinous growths that arise from the nasal mucosa and block the nasal and sinus passages. The cause of nasal polyps is unknown, but they appear to be the result of severe, prolonged inflammation that may be allergic or nonallergic.

In addition to obstructing the nasal passageway, polyps frequently produce a reduction in smell and taste, as well as postnasal drip. Occasionally, patients complain of facial pain and itchy eyes. Bronchial asthma is found in 30 percent of patients with nasal polyps.

Nasal Polyps and Asthma

An allergy to aspirin and related medications is a frequent finding in patients with both asthma and nasal polyps. It is estimated that as many as 20 percent of asthmatics are allergic or hypersensitive to aspirin. In these patients, aspirin produces a severe asthmatic attack. The hypersensitivity may not be manifested with the initial ingestion of aspirin, so a reaction may occur despite previous uncomplicated use of this drug. Because of this possibility, all asthmatics with nasal polyps should avoid aspirin.

A related group of medications called the nonsteroidal anti-inflammatory drugs (NSAIDs) may also produce asthmatic attacks in patients with asthma and nasal polyps. Many of this popular group of medications, such as ibuprofen and Naprosyn, are available without prescription. Patients with asthma and nasal polyps must be careful to avoid this group, as well as any cold medications that contain aspirin.

Diagnosis of Nasal Polyps

Nasal polyps are usually discovered during the physical examination. Many of the larger growths are visible with a simple examination of the nasal passage. Smaller lesions are often seen with the aid of the rhinoscope. Polyps may occur in the sinuses and be visualized on an x-ray or CAT scan.

Treatment of Nasal Polyps

Corticosteroids are often necessary for patients with severe obstruction of the nasal passage. This medication is usually initiated by mouth and slowly reduced, while a topical steroid spray is substituted. A topical spray may be sufficient in patients with milder symptoms.

Many patients with nasal polyps have sinus infections, so antibiotics may also be administered. In these patients, antibiotic therapy may be continued for as long as twenty-one days in order to eradicate the irritating infection.

SHOULD POLYPECTOMY BE PERFORMED?

When nasal polyps are large and the obstruction has not been decreased with medication, a polypectomy should be considered. This is usually a simple surgical procedure often performed in the outpatient setting. Patients with extensive sinus disease, however, may require a more significant procedure.

Unfortunately, nasal polyps have a high rate of recurrence. The use of a topical steroid spray after polypectomy, however, appears to decrease the chance of recurrence.

SLEEP APNEA

In the last decade, sleep apnea has been increasingly recognized as a disorder of breathing. It is now estimated that 5 percent of adult men suffer from sleep apnea, and as a consequence experience excessive daytime sleepiness (hypersomnolence). It is uncommon in women before menopause but occurs almost as frequently in postmenopausal women as in older men. Sleep apnea has also been described in children and adolescents and may occur at any age.

What Is Apnea?

Apnea is defined as an absence of air movement at the nose or mouth for at least ten seconds. More than 90 percent of sleep apneas occur due to a closure of the muscles of the upper respiratory tract (URT) and are called obstructive. These muscles support the throat and normally maintain the air-passage opening. When the muscles decrease their activity or tone, the passageway closes. In 10 percent of sleep apneas, these muscles do not produce closure of the upper air passage. These apneas are termed central because they appear to occur due to a malfunction in the brain's controlling centers.

Does Apnea Occur Normally?

Apnea is not always abnormal. Sleep studies have documented that adults may have as many as five apneas per hour. In patients with the sleep apnea syndrome, apneas occur more frequently and for longer time periods. In severe cases, the apneas may last for sixty to ninety seconds and may recur up to five hundred times in a night.

Obesity and Sleep Apnea

Most individuals with sleep apnea are overweight and many are obese. Obesity is defined by body weight that is 20 percent over the ideal predicted by age and sex. Although the relationship between obesity and sleep apnea is not clearly defined, the frequency of sleep-disordered breathing increases with weight gain. In many patients with the syndrome, improvement results from weight reduction.

Normal Sleep and Breathing

Normal sleep occurs in stages of decreased consciousness. In general, sleep can be divided into "quiet" or non-rapid eye movement sleep (non-REM) and "active" rapid eye movement sleep (REM). In adults, REM sleep accounts for 25 percent of sleep time. Most dreams occur during REM sleep, which may also exhibit twitching movements of the face and limbs.

During sleep, breathing becomes more shallow. As a result of the smaller breaths, oxygen levels decrease and carbon dioxide levels rise. The sensors located in the brain and carotid artery continue to respond to these changes but do so more slowly, particularly during REM sleep. In the normal individual, the smaller breaths and changes in blood gas levels during sleep have little physical effect. It has been demonstrated, however, that alcohol, tranquilizers, and sleeping pills exaggerate these changes and may severely depress breathing. In patients with breathing disorders, the change in breathing patterns during sleep may produce increased symptoms, as when oxygen levels fall. In these patients, oxygen may be administered during the hours of sleep.

Sleep Deprivation

Sleep deprivation has been shown to be detrimental to humans. Sleep, particularly REM sleep, appears to be essential for normal body function. Patients with obstructive sleep apnea (OSA) are sleep deprived due to a pattern of repeated apneas followed by awakening. A character-istic sequence of events is seen in OSA. The patient stops breathing while asleep and develops changes in blood gas levels. Arousal is pro-duced by the drop in blood oxygen levels and increase in carbon dioxide. He then falls asleep again and may repeat the cycle several times during the night. This severely fragmented sleep pattern produces excessive somnolence during the day. One of the consequences of daytime hyper-somnolence is a greater frequency of automobile accidents. Decreased productivity at work has also been documented.

Symptoms of Sleep Apnea:
The Snoring Man

Patients with OSA demonstrate symptoms while awake, as well as dur-ing sleep. The most helpful medical history on this disorder is obtained from a bed partner or family member. Individuals with OSA have little memory of what happens while they are sleeping.

The most common symptom of sleep apnea is snoring, which is caused by the fluttering of the soft tissue of the roof of the mouth. It is an important feature of OSA and is typically present for many years prior to diagnosis. It has been estimated that 45 percent of the normal population snores occasionally and 25 percent are habitual snorers. Snoring occurs more frequently in older men, but women after menopause snore almost as frequently. Obesity and heavy alcohol use are likely to increase snoring.

Nearly all patients with OSA snore. In these patients, snoring is irregular and interrupted by silences that end with loud grunting or gasping sounds. Snoring in OSA may reach noise levels that are haz-ardous to the bed partner's hearing. It is not uncommon for this person to sleep in another room to escape the noise.

As a pulmonary fellow on the Bellevue Chest Service, I was required to train for several months at the Manhattan Veterans Adminis-tration Hospital. Like many hospitals, the VA was divided into wards with patients often segregated by their diseases. It was on one of these wards that I heard "the snoring man."

One morning I was reviewing charts at one of the nurses' stations and became aware of a loud, rumbling noise emanating from somewhere on the ward. I swore later that the noise had vibrated the chart I was holding. Just when I would become curious about this sound, it would stop, only to start again in a minute or two. When I finally asked one of the nurses what the sound was, I was told it was "the snoring man." The snoring man was LG, a sixty-six-year-old veteran of World War II, who had been admitted with leg ulcers. He was 5 feet, 4 inches tall and weighed 275 pounds. I found him lying on several pillows in bed, fast asleep. His lips were blue, and just as I came close to him he stopped breathing. After twenty seconds he grunted loudly and awoke, saying, "I can't get any sleep." I introduced myself and as I started to question him, he fell asleep and began to snore. During this period his color had changed from a dusky purplish hue to pink. I had never seen a case of sleep apnea before and decided to return with some of my colleagues. As we entered, he was awakening with a start. "Do you know that you snore?" I asked him. "That's what they tell me, but I think they're making it up," he replied. A sleep study later documented that he had several hundred apneas during the night, some lasting as long as two minutes.

Patients with OSA may exhibit other symptoms during sleep. Fitfulness and flailing movements of the arms and legs are commonly observed. Sleepwalking and talking may occur in as many as 10 percent of patients.

During the day, the most common symptom of OSA is excessive sleepiness. Patients may awaken with a morning headache, which may be due to elevated carbon dioxide levels. They will often complain that sleep is not refreshing. Family members also complain about a change in the patient's personality, which may include uncharacteristic aggression and irritability. In children, symptoms of sleep apnea may be excessive daytime sleepiness, with decreased performance in school. Bed-wetting may also be noted.

Physical Findings of OSA

The most common physical finding of OSA is high blood pressure (hypertension). In one study of patients with OSA, 96 percent were hypertensive. The source of elevated blood pressure is thought to be due to stimulation of the nervous system and lowered oxygen levels. It has been estimated that undiagnosed OSA may occur in as many as 40 percent of all patients with high blood pressure.

Approximately 40 percent of patients with OSA are obese. Patients with severe OSA may exhibit physical findings that reflect severe derangements in blood gas levels. When oxygen falls and carbon dioxide rises, there is a reflex mechanism that produces increased work of the right side of the heart. Pressure in the lung's blood vessels also increases. If the blood-gas abnormalities are sustained, the heart muscle may weaken and result in heart failure. These patients often demonstrate cyanosis, the bluish discoloration of the skin that occurs with low oxygen levels. The weakened heart is unable to pump normally, which causes fluid retention. This is manifested by swelling of the legs and abdomen. These patients with severe OSA often complain of shortness of breath due to the low oxygen levels. Many of these patients require oxygen during the day, as well as while sleeping. It should be remembered, however, that patients with OSA often do not have any symptoms.

CHECKING THE UVULA

In patients with OSA, it is important to examine the throat. This area is known to close in patients with OSA. A structural narrowing of the upper airway may be occasionally noted. One simple example is enlarged tonsils. The fleshy extension of the soft palate, which hangs down at the back of the mouth, is called the uvula. In some patients, an abnormally long uvula has been implicated in OSA.

The Sleep Study

Although patients may present with characteristic symptoms of sleep apnea, as well as the noted physical findings, a formal sleep study is required for diagnosis. Sleep studies, called polysomnography, are usually performed at special centers according to standardized guidelines. A typical study is performed overnight with monitoring of brain activity, airflow, EKG, and oxygen levels. Once sleep apnea has been documented, patients often return for evaluation of treatment options.

The Treatment of Sleep Apnea

In view of the fact that apneas can occur normally, treatment depends on the severity of the symptoms and the presence of significant complications, such as a low oxygen level. Patients who lack symptoms may not require treatment.

Patients with sleep apnea are advised to avoid alcohol, tranquilizers, and sleeping pills, since these substances depress breathing and may aggravate the condition. In obese patients, weight reduction may dramatically reduce the number and severity of the apneas. In some patients, a loss of 5 to 10 percent of body weight produces marked improvement. Unfortunately, the effect of weight reduction is unpredictable.

An interesting mode of treatment of sleep apnea is the adjustment of the position or posture in which the patient sleeps. Sleep apnea is often worse when sleeping on the back. The frequency and duration of apneas may be decreased by sleeping on the side. Sleep-position training is accomplished by a number of innovative techniques. One is to sew a tennis ball into the back of a nightshirt so that it will be uncomfortable to sleep in the supine position.

Several medications have been tried in patients with sleep apnea without consistently beneficial results. Examples include the female hormone progesterone and the bronchodilator theophylline. These drugs have a stimulatory effect on breathing. Unfortunately, the results of these and other medications have been disappointing.

NASAL CPAP

The most effective form of treatment for OSA is the application of continuous positive airway pressure (nasal CPAP). In OSA, the muscles of the throat relax, which results in closure of the air passageway. In nasal CPAP, a force of air is applied in the form of a small, tight-fitting plastic mask that fits over the nose. The air passes through the nasal passages and, in effect, acts like a splint for the upper airway. The amount of pressure must be carefully adjusted for each patient. This is usually done with a repeat sleep study to document reduction in the number and severity of the apneas. This device is now commercially available and covered by most insurance plans.

After receiving nasal CPAP therapy for a short time, improvement in the condition may eliminate the need for nightly treatment. Symptoms reappear, however, if nasal CPAP is completely withdrawn. The primary drawback of this form of treatment is the restriction in movement that it requires, as well as nasal discomfort. Some patients require nasal decongestants or topical steroid sprays to maintain the opening of the nasal passages. Five to 30 percent of patients with OSA are unable to tolerate nasal CPAP on a long-term basis.

Is There a Place for Surgery?

A surgical approach to the problem of OSA may be applicable to selected patients. When there is severe nasal obstruction due to a deviated septum or nasal polyps, for example, nasal surgery to restore the passageway may be helpful.

A relatively new procedure called uvulopalatopharyngoplasty (UPPP) has proved helpful in a number of patients. This procedure enlarges the upper airway by removing excess tissue from the pharynx. Results suggest that this procedure is most useful in patients who clearly have a long, redundant soft palate that narrows the upper airway. One study demonstrated a success rate of 45 percent in patients with OSA.

ASTHMA

Asthma is a chronic disease of the air passages of the lung that affects nearly 5 percent of the population in the United States, perhaps as many as fifteen million people. Since asthma is often a mild illness, these numbers probably underestimate the true number of cases. Asthma is the most common chronic disease of childhood, affecting an estimated 4.8 million children. Between 1982 and 1992, the asthma rate increased by 42 percent, attributed partly to air pollution, since the majority of asthmatics live in areas where air-pollution levels are high. Indoor pollution may also be a factor because windowless offices and airtight homes reduce air circulation, thus exposing asthmatics to higher levels of irritating substances.

Despite newer and better drugs, more than five thousand people die of asthma each year. Each of these deaths is tragic, since in most cases fatal attacks can be prevented. Death rates have been consistently highest among blacks and children. These rates have increased or remained stable over the past decade.

What Is Asthma?

Asthma is defined as a chronic inflammatory disorder of the air passages, or bronchial tubes. Inflammation is a response to injury or stimulation that produces redness, swelling, and warmth. In asthma, the lining of the bronchial tubes appears red and swollen. In susceptible individuals, this inflammation produces episodes of breathlessness, wheezing, chest tightness, and cough, particularly at night and in the early morning.

In asthma, bronchial tubes become narrowed or constricted. This is called airway obstruction because air can no longer flow smoothly through this elaborate system of branching tubes. Since these passages can dilate or open in asthma, this obstruction is called reversible, an important feature of this illness because it may distinguish asthma from other bronchial disorders—bronchitis or emphysema—with fixed or irreversible obstruction.

Another important characteristic of asthma is a tendency to overreact to various stimuli. This feature is called hyperresponsiveness and is demonstrated by the sudden, severe attacks asthmatics may experience when exposed to substances such as pollen, animal dander, dust, and fumes.

What Causes Asthma?

Although asthma's exact cause remains unknown, research has identified several important factors that may produce this condition.

HEREDITY

Heredity plays a major role: Asthma and allergy often occur in families. Geneticists have located several genes that are directly associated with allergy and asthma. One of these genes directs the immune system to overreact to allergic stimuli by producing Immunoglobulin E (IgE), which "locks on" to the surface of mast cells. When IgE reacts with allergy substances, the mast cell disintegrates, releasing irritating chemicals that cause inflammation. The genetic predisposition to produce IgE and this reaction is the strongest identifiable predisposing factor for developing asthma.

THE IMMUNE SYSTEM

The immune system also plays a major role in the development of asthma. The immune system has two basic branches: cellular and humoral. Cellular immunity involves white blood cells, called lymphocytes, which can be provoked or "sensitized." Humoral immunity involves the production of substances called antibodies, which circulate in the blood. An antigen (may be called an allergen) is a substance capable of provoking the immune response.

Lymphocytes, Neutrophils, and Eosinophils

In asthma, the immune system is provoked in two ways. First, the cellular elements are mobilized. Microscopic studies of the lining of the bronchial tubes in asthma have revealed increased numbers of inflammatory cells. Many of these cells are lymphocytes. They produce substances that result in an increase in the number of mast cells, which are known to store and release many irritating chemicals involved in the production of the asthmatic reaction. These chemical substances, or mediators, of asthma produce inflammation. Another active cell that is "recruited" by lymphocytes found in the inflamed bronchial lining is the eosinophil. Large numbers of these cells may also be found in the blood of allergic and asthmatic individuals. Another white blood cell, called a neutrophil, has been seen in inflamed bronchial linings. Many of these cells are often noted in sudden, fatal asthmatic attacks.

ALLERGY

Allergy is the leading cause of asthma. Allergens, activated lymphocytes, mast cells, eosinophils, and IgE all play major roles in the immune response that produces the asthmatic reaction. However, asthma may also occur without allergy. In nonallergic patients, doctors believe the immune response may be triggered by infection.

VIRUSES

Viral infections in susceptible individuals have been thought to be potent triggers for the development of asthma. Animal research has shown that viruses are capable of altering the nervous impulses that stimulate the bronchial tubes. The altered nerve impulses may then produce constriction in the bronchial tubes. Susceptible individuals with viral bronchial infections may become sensitized and display all the noted characteristics of asthma.

THE ENVIRONMENT

Environmental irritants, such as cigarette smoke, air pollutants (ozone, particulates, sulfur dioxide, nitrogen dioxide), dust, and chemicals and proteins found in the home and the workplace are also considered capable of provoking the asthmatic response. These irritants account for large numbers of asthmatic attacks each year and may also, in part, explain an increase in the number of asthma cases.

How Is the Diagnosis of Asthma Made?

THE MEDICAL HISTORY

The medical history may provide important information that leads to the diagnosis of asthma. The physician looks for the age at onset of symptoms and associated allergies. Evidence of airway obstruction may be suggested by a report of wheezing and shortness of breath. Coughing may be a prominent symptom, and the physician will inquire as to the character of phlegm (sputum) produced. The physician will also ask about the presence of nasal or sinus symptoms, as well as the presence of allergic skin problems, such as rash (eczema) or hives (urticaria). Common questions include: "What seems to trigger your attack?" "What are your attacks like?" Asthma is often worse at night and the patient may be asked, "Do you ever awaken with an attack?"

The timing of attacks other than at night is also important. A relationship between asthma and hormonal influences should be explored. Many women note increased asthmatic symptoms before their periods, as well as changes during pregnancy. The physician will ask about the effect of exercise on the patient's symptoms. Emotional factors will also be investigated as potential triggers: "Are you under more stress?" A thorough family history will also be obtained, since the presence of asthma or allergy in closely related family members supports the diagnosis. An occupational history is also important as asthma may be produced by exposure to irritating chemicals, dust, or fumes. To help establish the hyperresponsiveness evident in asthma, the physician will ask how the patient reacts to changes in temperature, humidity, air pollution, or the presence of cigarette smoke, fumes, or odors. Reaction to foods containing sulfites, as well as to drugs (especially aspirin and penicillin) are also important historical factors.

THE PHYSICAL EXAMINATION

The physical exam may add important information that contributes to the diagnosis of asthma. Examination of the skin and nasal passages may identify allergic conditions, such as eczema and rhinitis. As noted previously, the finding of nasal polyps identifies the patient as someone who may have severe allergy or asthma.

In examining the chest, the physician will note the quality of the breathing sounds as air is inhaled and exhaled. When there is airway obstruction, the flow of air through the bronchial tubes is turbulent and often creates wheezing, which is more commonly noted upon exhaling. In addition, the narrowed passages prolong the time it takes for air to be exhaled. Although the patient's breathing may be quiet at rest, when asked to take a deep breath and exhale, wheezing and coughing may occur, which enables a physician to discover airway obstruction.

Asthma without Wheezing ("Cough Asthma")

In the past decade, it has become clear that a group of patients with all of the characteristics of asthma (inflammation, airway obstruction, hyperresponsiveness) may never manifest wheezing. A persistent cough is the main symptom in these patients. Although the physical exam may be unremarkable, these patients often have typical histories of cough attacks at night or when triggered by exposure to allergens. This syndrome is often identified as "cough asthma" or the asthma equivalent syndrome. In the past, too much weight has been put on the presence of wheezing in the diagnosis of asthma.

Wheezing without Asthma

Just as the absence of wheezing has often led to patients being misdiagnosed as nonasthmatic, the *presence* of wheezing also may lead to the erroneous diagnosis of asthma. It has been said that "all that wheezes is not asthma," as many illnesses may produce turbulent airflow through the airways. Too often, patients are diagnosed simply based on this one physical finding.

Wheezing may occur in a variety of illnesses. In a child or an adult, this may be as simple as a foreign body that has been aspirated. In these cases, wheezing may be localized to one area or one lung, which should alert the physician to this possibility. Wheezing may be a prominent finding in lung cancer, emphysema, and chronic bronchitis.

"CARDIAC ASTHMA"

Fluid may collect in the lungs around or within the bronchial tubes of patients with heart failure. These patients often complain of shortness of breath and wheezing, especially at night, mimicking the asthma patient. Because of the similarity of features, this has been called cardiac asthma, although it is a heart syndrome. The diagnosis is often made after additional physical findings of heart disease, as well as by the chest x-ray and other tests of heart function.

LARYNGEAL ASTHMA

A rare but increasingly reported illness that produces wheezing and may be misdiagnosed as asthma is vocal cord dysfunction syndrome. It is also known as laryngeal asthma because in this illness wheezing is produced at the voice box by an abnormal closure of the vocal cords when the patient inhales. Normally, the vocal cords separate on inspiration, allowing more air to flow into the lungs. In these patients, the sounds of turbulent flow are transmitted over the lung fields, mimicking the wheezing of asthma. The disorder's cause is unknown. It is thought to be involuntary and often responds to voice therapy. The diagnosis may only be made by direct visualization of the vocal cords by the physician.

Laboratory Evaluation of Asthma

The laboratory evaluation of asthma will include blood tests to assess allergy, plain chest x-ray, and pulmonary function testing. Allergy skin testing is only recommended for patients with more severe or persistent symptoms.

The chest x-ray primarily eliminates the possibility of other chest diseases, since the bronchial tubes are not easily seen via this technique. Occasionally, the chest x-ray may show that the lungs are greatly expanded and appear larger than normal (hyperinflated). This occurs in asthma because air may enter the bronchial tubes but have difficulty being exhaled, also known as air trapping. This may also be seen in emphysema and bronchitis so it cannot be used to diagnose asthma.

PULMONARY FUNCTION TESTING

The most important laboratory test that the physician performs in the diagnosis of asthma is pulmonary function testing. (See Chapter 2.)

Spirometry

By performing spirometry before and after the inhalation of a bronchodilator medication, the physician establishes the presence of reversible airway obstruction. However, it may be difficult to demonstrate reversibility in all asthmatics during a single laboratory session, possibly owing to severe degrees of bronchial narrowing or to a patient's inadequate inhalation of medication. Therefore, the absence of reversibility should never be taken as absolute proof that asthma is not present.

Bronchial Challenge Testing

In some asthmatics, spirometry may be normal. In patients with typical symptoms that prompt the physician to strongly suspect asthma, a challenge test may be done. This is not part of routine pulmonary function testing.

Bronchial challenge testing is done with a variety of substances that the patient inhales under controlled conditions. These substances include cold air and chemicals such as histamine, which may trigger the asthmatic reaction. A positive result means there is at least a 15 percent reduction in airflows after inhaling the challenge material.

Measuring Peak Flow

Asthmatics may participate in their care by performing a home measurement called peak flow. This is not unlike the diabetic who monitors blood sugar to determine proper treatment.

Peak flow is the maximum airflow an individual can generate with forced expiration. It is one of the measurements that the spirometer records, but it can also be measured with a simple handheld flowmeter. This inexpensive device can serve as an early warning system for patients with asthma, as well as provide invaluable information for the physician.

Peak flow meters have moved into the electronic age in the form of a device known as AirWatch, which is manufactured by Enact. (See the appendix.) In addition to recording and storing much more information than the simple flowmeter, it can transfer its data over the phone lines to the physician.

The Treatment of Bronchial Asthma

The treatment of bronchial asthma combines the avoidance of known allergens and irritants with the administration of appropriate medication. In most cases, these medications focus on reversing both the constriction of the bronchial tubes and inflammation within them.

AVOIDANCE

Avoidance of allergens has been largely discussed in the treatment of allergic rhinitis. This is another area in which patients can take an active role in their care by allergy-proofing their homes, cars, and offices. In many cases, patients may identify specific "triggers" of their attacks and then eliminate these substances from their environments.

Cigarette Smoking

Patients with asthma who smoke do not have far to look to find a reason to stop. Cigarette smoking is the leading cause of respiratory illness and death in the United States. All of these illnesses and deaths are preventable. Cigarette smoking may increase the "irritability" of the bronchial tubes and may directly trigger an asthmatic attack. Smoking also affects the immune response and the lung's defense mechanisms against infection. Smokers have higher rates of sinus and bronchial infections than do nonsmokers. These infections may also trigger asthmatic attacks.

Despite these facts and the tremendous amount of evidence demonstrating a cause-and-effect relationship between smoking and lung cancer, as well as emphysema and heart disease, many patients with asthma continue to smoke. Some stop during attacks and resume when they feel better.

Environmental Tobacco Smoke

Nonsmokers are exposed to many of the same injurious agents inhaled by active smokers. The dangers of secondhand tobacco smoke have been widely publicized. (See Table 3.3.) It should be noted that children exposed to parental secondhand smoke have been found to have more respiratory illnesses, including asthma. Asthmatic children of smokers

TABLE 3.3 THE EFFECTS OF SECONDHAND SMOKE

Disease	Annual cases or deaths in United States
Asthma in children	8,000–26,000 new cases 400,000 to 1 million flare-ups of existing cases
Bronchitis in children	150,000–300,000 cases
Lung cancer	3,000 deaths
Sudden infant death syndrome	1,900–2,700 cases
Low–birth weight babies	9,700–18,600 cases

have been shown to have more frequent attacks. Environmental tobacco smoke is one the most frequently reported triggers of asthmatic attacks.

Wood Smoke and Gas Stoves

Wood smoke from wood-burning stoves and fireplaces may also be an irritant and aggravate bronchial asthma. Approximately 6 percent of homes in the United States have wood stoves, and 19 percent have fireplaces. Although the smoke from wood stoves and fireplaces is vented to the outdoors, emissions are found to contaminate indoor air during start-up and stoking. Particulate matter may also be produced by these sources and irritate bronchial asthma.

Gas stoves may also be a source of indoor pollution. Several airborne irritants may be released by gas combustion, including nitrogen dioxide. As a rule, asthmatics should avoid gas and wood-burning stoves.

Cockroaches

A recent study of asthma cases occurring in a large city found a strong connection between allergy to cockroaches and the number of asthmatic attacks. The increased frequency of asthma, as well as asthma deaths, has been seen in predominantly inner-city residents. All asthmatics should be aware of this potential allergy, and if cockroaches are present in their homes, invoke control measures, including control of sources of food and water, routine cleaning, and regular use of insecticides, such as hydramethylnon and avermectin, in the form of bait.

Air Temperature

Patients should also consider air temperature. Cold air is irritating in asthmatics and may produce severe attacks. Individuals with asthma appear to warm air less quickly and efficiently than do non-asthmatics. One simple measure patients should take is to wrap their faces with a scarf that warms the air before it is inhaled. A cold-air mask is commercially available and may provide more protection in the winter. (See the appendix.)

The Asthma Diet

Patients with asthma can also participate in their care by monitoring their diets. Asthmatics who have experienced allergic reactions to specific foods must carefully avoid these products. Reactions may include the development of hives (urticaria), wheezing, collapse of the circulation, and swelling of the throat (anaphylaxis). Common causes of allergic or asthmatic reactions include shrimp and other shellfish, eggs, milk, soy, and peanuts. Asthma attacks triggered by food allergies are much more common in children, particularly those with an allergic skin rash known as eczema.

A recent study has suggested that a diet rich in magnesium may benefit lung function and may actually reduce wheezing and bronchial irritability. Magnesium is found in cereals, nuts, green vegetables, and dairy products.

Sulfites

Sulfites are a common food and beverage preservative that may cause asthmatic attacks in sensitive individuals. These preservatives have been used to make products appear fresh and reduce spoilage. This practice and the resulting asthmatic attacks have led to the use of the term *restaurant asthma*. It is believed that the irritant producing the asthmatic reaction is sulfur dioxide gas liberated from salts of sulfite, bisulfite, or metabisulfite.

Some of the products containing sulfites that may cause reactions include processed potatoes, baked products, fresh shrimp, fruit drinks, dried fruits, beer, and wine. Sulfites have also been used as preservatives in medications, including some asthma medications that are used in nebulizers. Sulfite-free nebulizer solutions are now widely available.

THE ASTHMA MEDICATIONS

Asthma medications are often divided into "controllers" and "relievers." Relievers include short-acting bronchodilating medications that act quickly to relieve the constriction of the bronchial tubes and the accompanying symptoms, such as cough, chest tightness, and wheezing. The controllers are taken daily on a long-term basis and represent the anti-inflammatory medications and long-acting bronchodilators.

The Bronchodilators

Preferred: The Beta-Agonists

The most effective bronchodilators for the treatment of asthma are the B_2-adrenergic agonists. These medications are all derivatives of epinephrine, which affects the heart (termed beta-1) and lung (beta-2). Epinephrine is an important hormone produced in the body by the adrenal gland but has been synthesized in the laboratory. The B_2-adrenergic agonists have been developed to be "selective" stimulants of lung receptors. One such B_2-receptor is located in the muscle layer that surrounds the bronchial tube. With the administration of these agents and stimulation of the receptor, the bronchial wall muscle relaxes, producing bronchodilatation.

For the Acute Asthmatic Attack: Short-Acting Agents

Several selective B_2-adrenergic agonists are available for use. These agents are available as aerosol sprays delivered by metered-dose inhalers (MDIs); aerosol solution to be delivered by nebulization; dry powder for inhalation (DPI); short- and long-acting tablets; and as flavored syrups for children.

In the acute asthmatic attack, the treatment of choice for prompt relief of symptoms is the administration of a short-acting B_2-adrenergic agonist. B_2-adrenergic agonists (albuterol, metaproterenol, pirbuterol, terbutaline, fenoterol, and bitolterol) have a rapid onset of action (within minutes) with a duration of action of four to six hours. The recommended dosage is two puffs every six hours as needed. These medications differ in potency, as well as in how fast they begin to work, and when their peak effect is reached. Table 3.4 lists the B_2-agonists by generic and brand name, as well as the types of preparations that are available.

Long-Acting B₂-Agonists

Longer-acting B_2-adrenergic agonists (salmeterol, formoterol) delivered by a metered-dose inhaler have been developed, with a duration of action of up to twelve hours. These medications are used for maintenance therapy.

Salmeterol. Salmeterol is the only long-acting B_2-adrenergic agonist that is available in the United States. The recommended dosage is two puffs every twelve hours administered on a regular basis. When compared with albuterol, salmeterol is more potent and more selective. A dry powder preparation, called Serevent Diskus, has recently become available in the United States.

TABLE 3.4 THE B₂-ADRENERGIC AGONISTS

Drug Name	Brand Name	Preparations	Comments
Albuterol	Proventil, Ventolin	MDI, DPI, tablet, nebulizer, syrup	Selective, short to medium duration
Bitolterol	Tornalate	MDI, nebulizer	Selective
Isoetharine	Bronkosol, Bronkometer	MDI, nebulizer	Selective, short duration
Fenoterol	Berotec	MDI	Selective, not available in USA
Metaproterenol	Alupent, Metaprel	MDI, nebulizer, tablet, syrup	Less selective
Pirbuterol	Maxair	MDI, Autohaler	Selective
Salmeterol	Serevent	MDI, DPI (Serevent Diskus)	Selective, long duration
Terbutaline	Brethaire, Brethine, Bricanyl	MDI, injection, tablets	Selective, DPI available in Europe

The longer-acting B_2-agonists are particularly helpful as maintenance therapy for moderate asthma and in the prevention of nocturnal asthmatic attacks. Patients wake up with better peak flows and have fewer flare-ups of their asthma. The twice-a-day administration provides greater convenience for the patient. Note, however, that the onset of action of the long-acting B_2-agonists is thirty to forty-five minutes. In view of this delayed onset, the long-acting B_2-agonists should not be used for relief of an acute asthmatic attack.

Delivering the Bronchodilator: Aerosol Therapy

The fastest and most effective method of administering a bronchodilator is by inhalation. An asthma aerosol is a mixture of a liquid medication suspended in a gas that can be inhaled. Aerosols differ in the size of the spray or mist particles that are inhaled. Examples of asthma aerosols are sprays from metered-dose inhalers and nebulizers.

Metered-Dose Inhalers

A metered-dose inhaler contains a medication suspended in a mixture of a liquid propellant gas and preservatives. This mixture is contained in a metal canister that sits in a plastic shell. When downward pressure is applied to the canister, the medication mixture passes through a valve and is transformed under pressure into a fine spray that can be inhaled. The propellant used in most MDIs is a mixture of freon gases called chlorofluorocarbons (CFCs). Although safe to inhale, CFCs are damaging to the atmosphere and destroy its protective ozone layer. The Montreal Protocol, an international agreement reached in 1987, calls for the replacement of CFC inhalers by the year 2000. This process has already begun with the introduction of alternative propellants (HFA-134a, HFA-227). At least one non-CFC MDI is now available (Proventil-HFA) and more will follow until all CFC sprays have been phased out.

The MDI is a compact and portable device that rapidly dispenses a certain amount of medication. Coordination between hand activation of the MDI and breathing must exist if the medication is to be delivered properly. Instruction in the use of an MDI is important in order to maximize the amount of medication reaching the lungs. (See Fig. 3.2.)

Spacers

Patients who experience difficulty with metered-dose inhalers may benefit from the use of a spacer or extension tube. Spacers come in different sizes (large or small volume) and shapes. In its simplest form, a spacer consists of an attachment that fits over the MDI's mouthpiece.

How to Use a Metered-Dose Inhaler

1. Shake the inhaler well.
2. Exhale fully (empty your lungs).
3. Place the mouthpiece an inch in front of the open mouth ("open-mouth technique"). Make sure the inhaler is in the upright position.
4. While inhaling slowly and deeply through the mouth, use your index finger to fully depress the top of the canister.
5. Hold your breath at least ten seconds.
6. Relax, wait one minute before taking another spray.
7. **Note:** In the "closed-mouth technique," step 3 requires that the MDI mouthpiece be placed fully into the mouth, with the lips closed around it.

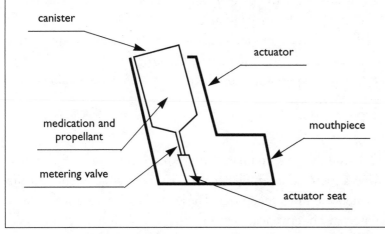

canister

actuator

medication and propellant

mouthpiece

metering valve

actuator seat

FIG. 3.2 DIAGRAM OF METERED-DOSE INHALER AND INSTRUCTIONS ON ITS USE.

Activation of the inhaler allows the medication to enter the attached chamber from which the patient then inhales. Use of this device improves delivery of medication and reduces the amount lost in the mouth and throat.

Although the amount of medication deposited and lost in the mouth may be reduced by even the simplest spacer, it appears that the larger-volume spacers are more effective than the smaller devices.

The total body absorption of inhaled medication is greatly influenced by the amount deposited in the mouth. This material makes up the highest proportion of medication that is absorbed. By reducing the amount lost in the mouth, spacers reduce total-body absorption and may therefore reduce possible total-body side effects. This benefit may be particularly advantageous in the use of the topical corticosteroid sprays.

Nebulizers

A nebulizer may also be used to rapidly deliver aerosol medication. This device, which is commonly found in an emergency room setting, is basically a simple system that allows rapidly flowing air or oxygen to be bubbled through a solution containing the medication. This system produces a medicated mist the patient inhales. Nebulizers differ in terms of the size of the particles they produce.

Nebulizer delivery of a bronchodilator is preferred in the emergency room setting because a larger amount of the drug can be delivered. The nebulizer does not require the coordination between hand and breathing necessary for MDI use.

Better Than MDI?

Several studies have compared the effectiveness of a B_2-agonist delivered by a metered-dose inhaler with a spacer attachment and the same drug delivered by a nebulizer. These studies have shown little or no difference in effectiveness between the two delivery systems, perhaps because a metered-dose spray enables the patient to take a deep breath to deliver the bronchodilator medication, while with a nebulizer, the patient breathes normally. The deep breath may be advantageous to the delivery of medication to smaller bronchial tubes. During a severe attack, however, it may be difficult for patients to inhale deeply enough, so that greater benefit is achieved with a nebulizer.

▒ Dry Powder Inhalers: The Future?

Dry powder inhalers (DPIs) provide an alternative method for the administration of medication by inhalation. With the phasing out of CFC-containing MDIs, it is likely that the number of medications available in DPI form will increase. Two B_2-adrenergic agonists, albuterol (Ventolin Rotohaler), and salmeterol (Serevent Diskus), are available in this form.

DPIs were originally manufactured to dispense a single dose of medication at a time, requiring reloading between each use. This type of device has not proven to be popular in this country. More sophisticated multidose dispensers, containing thirty or more doses, have been widely used in Europe and were recently introduced here (Serevent Diskus, Pulmicort).

Dry powder inhalers may be particularly helpful for patients who have difficulty using MDIs, since coordination between the hand and breathing is unnecessary. With a DPI, the device is breath activated. It is important for the patient's lips to be tightly sealed around the mouthpiece and to inhale slowly and deeply.

Patients who experience severe asthmatic attacks may have difficulty generating adequate airflow to deliver the full amount of medication from a DPI. When this kind of attack occurs, these patients should receive bronchodilator medication delivered by an MDI with a spacer or with the use of a nebulizer. It is likely that in the future, this problem will be overcome by the development of a battery-powered DPI that generates the force required to propel the medication.

▒ Second-Line Agent: Theophylline

Theophylline has been used for treating asthma for nearly sixty years but is a weaker bronchodilator than the B_2-adrenergic agonists and should be considered a second choice. Although widely used as a bronchodilator, the mechanism of its action is unclear. The most recent information suggests an anti-inflammatory effect.

Theophylline is an oral medication, which may be preferred by some patients who do not tolerate the B_2-agonists or have difficulty using aerosol sprays. It is available in a time-release form that permits dosing on a once- or twice-a-day schedule. Theophylline has been helpful in preventing nocturnal asthmatic attacks and is often given in the evening. When theophylline is given by mouth, an effect may be achieved in approximately one hour, but it may require two to three days to achieve the desired maintenance blood level. Laboratory testing permits the measurement of the amount of this medication in the blood.

One drawback to theophylline is that a certain amount must be given in order to achieve an effect. This has been termed a therapeutic level (10 to 20 milligrams of the drug per liter of blood). Some patients, however, may benefit from lower levels. Once a patient is started on theophylline, blood levels should be performed to determine if the therapeutic level has been reached.

Compared with the rapidly acting B_2-agonists, theophylline is both weaker and slower in producing bronchodilatation. Theophylline also has a greater incidence of adverse effects, which include stomach and bowel upset, rapid or irregular heartbeat, insomnia, nervousness, urinary frequency, and headache. Some of these side effects may be prevented or reduced by avoiding caffeine, which is structurally similar to theophylline, which explains why coffee has often been noted to relieve asthma.

Second-Line Agent: The Anticholinergics

For thousands of years, it has been observed that anticholinergic drugs had beneficial effects on many patients with respiratory diseases. In fact, many ancient herbal preparations have been found to include atropine (from leaves of the *Atropa belladonna* plant) and stramonium (from the plant *Datura stramonium*). Stramonium cigarettes were commonly smoked in the late nineteenth century for the relief of asthma.

How Anticholinergic Drugs Work

The action of the anticholinergic agent is believed to be primarily on the tone of the bronchial wall muscle. This muscle tone is thought to be controlled in part by the vagus nerve, a component of the nervous pathway called the cholinergic nervous system. Cholinergic receptors coexist in the bronchial wall muscle with the adrenergic receptors. When the cholinergic receptor is stimulated, the activity of the vagus nerve is reduced, resulting in relaxation of the bronchial wall muscle and bronchodilatation.

In bronchial asthma, the role of the cholinergic system is minor and therefore the effects of anticholinergic drugs are weak compared with B-adrenergic agonists. Anticholinergic agents, however, are of greater value for patients with emphysema and chronic bronchitis where it is clear that vagal cholinergic tone plays a greater role.

Ipratropium Bromide

Ipratropium bromide (Atrovent) is available as an aerosol medication for metered-dose inhalers and in solution for nebulization. The recommended MDI dose is two puffs every six hours. Ipratropium bromide has a slow onset of action, which may not peak for sixty minutes. Adverse effects are few and include headache and a bitter taste. Patients with narrow-angle glaucoma and enlargement of the prostate gland should avoid it.

Anti-Inflammatory Drugs

With greater emphasis being placed on the inflammatory nature of asthma, the anti-inflammatory agents have achieved greater importance in treatment.

Inhaled Corticosteroids

The most potent and effective anti-inflammatory agents are corticosteroids, limited to oral or injectable forms until relatively recently, when an inhalation form became available. The "topically active" inhaled steroids have radically changed and improved the treatment of bronchial asthma.

The inhaled corticosteroids (beclomethasone dipropionate, triamcinolone acetonide, flunisolide, budesonide, fluticasone) are topically active and achieve their effect on the surface of the bronchial lining. Compared with the B-adrenergic agonists, corticosteroids do not have an immediate effect and cannot rapidly reduce symptoms, which is why patients may stop this important medication before it has had an adequate trial. Remember that the primary purpose of corticosteroid sprays is prevention. If used correctly, these agents may provide long-term control over asthma.

Specific Agents

Table 3.5 lists the inhaled corticosteroids, their brand names, and the forms that are available. These agents may be given in varying dosages depending on individual patients. A common starting dose would be 400 micrograms (μg) per day given in divided doses morning and night.

TABLE 3.5 INHALED CORTICOSTEROIDS

Drug	Brand Name	Strength μg/Puff	Form	Comments
Beclomethasone dipropionate	Vanceril, Vanceril DS	42 84	MDI	High dose (250) (Becloforte) and DPI (Becotide, Becodisks) available in Canada, Europe
Budesonide	Pulmicort	200	DPI	MDI and 50, 400 strength available in Canada, Europe
Flunisolide	Aerobid	250	MDI	Mint flavor form, Aerobid-M
Fluticasone propionate	Flovent Rotadisk	44, 110, 220 50, 100, 250	MDI DPI	MDI and DPI available in 3 dosages
Triamcinolone acetonide	Azmacort	100	MDI	Incorporates spacer device

Adverse Effects and How to Prevent Them

In general, inhaled corticosteroids are well tolerated and safe at the recommended dosages. The small risk of adverse effects is well balanced by their effectiveness. The primary side effect of inhaled corticosteroids is development of a yeast infection, known as candidiasis, in the mouth or throat. This is a local infection and the rare instances of its spreading outside the mouth have typically occurred in patients with lowered immunity, who took no precautionary steps. Several preventive measures can be taken to avoid the infection, including rinsing the mouth (and spitting) after spraying. Another helpful step in administering inhaled steroids aimed at reducing the risk of yeast infection is a spacer. This simple device that attaches to the MDI improves delivery of the steroid to the lung, as well as reduces the amount likely to be deposited in the mouth and throat.

Another infrequent side effect of inhaled steroids is an effect on the voice. This uncommon result is usually noted as hoarseness and may be alleviated with a spacer and by temporary reduction in dosage.

Are There Total-Body Effects?

Many patients fear that inhaled corticosteroids will produce total-body effects similar to those produced by taking steroids by mouth or injection. Recent reports have demonstrated a higher incidence of cataracts and glaucoma in patients using inhaled steroids. In general, inhaled steroids are not absorbed in appreciable amounts into the bloodstream and total body. The use of high dosages of these agents for a prolonged period, however, may produce a greater risk of total-body effects. Whenever possible, maintenance dosages should be reduced to 400 micrograms per day or less.

Recent research has demonstrated that the combination of a long-acting B_2-agonist (salmeterol, formoterol) with low doses of a topical corticosteroid produces benefits that are greater to or equal to high doses of a topical steroid spray alone. The combination of theophylline with low doses of a topical steroid has also been found to be equal in benefit to the effect of high doses of the steroid spray. These studies indicate that high doses of a topical corticosteroid spray can frequently be avoided and the risk of side effects reduced.

Systemic Corticosteroids

Before the introduction of inhaled corticosteroids in the 1970s, these agents were limited to oral and injectable preparations that produced total-body or systemic effects. Many patients with asthma became steroid dependent for life and developed serious side effects. Although inhaled corticosteroids have spared many patients this "life sentence" or allowed many to reduce their steroid dosages, systemic corticosteroids are still often required to treat acute and severe asthma.

In patients with severe attacks who are already receiving bronchodilator and anti-inflammatory therapy, a course of an oral steroid such as prednisone, prednisolone, or methylprednisolone will be necessary. Those patients who require emergency room care and/or hospitalization often also require intravenous preparations of hydrocortisone (Solucortef) or methylprednisolone (Solumedrol).

Considering the Adrenal Gland

The adrenal gland produces the body's own supply of cortisone. When this gland recognizes that corticosteroid is present in the bloodstream in quantities greater than usual, it stops its own production. This is called adrenal suppression, and the state of inactivity is termed adrenal insufficiency. In this state, the absence of cortisone under stressful conditions may produce low blood pressure and shock. Because of this effect on the adrenal gland, once systemic steroids are administered, they are usually tapered off rather than stopped abruptly. Patients who have been steroid dependent for prolonged periods must be carefully monitored when systemic steroids are withdrawn.

Adverse Effects of Systemic Steroids

Any adverse effects of corticosteroids are directly related to how long they are administered and in what dosage. The greater the dosage the more likely the development of side effects, especially if sustained at high dosage for a prolonged period (months to years). One of the most serious side effects is the development of adrenal insufficiency. Other adverse effects include high blood pressure, diabetes, stomach ulcer, osteoporosis, mental changes, fluid retention, thinning of the skin with easy bruising, accelerated cataract formation, irregular periods, and obesity.

Preparing for Side Effects

When corticosteroids are prescribed, it is best to prepare for side effects, including careful monitoring of caloric intake, salt, and fluid consumed in an attempt to reduce weight gain and swelling. Increased exercise can help slow weight gains. Exercise is important because steroids may cause myopathy, or muscle weakness. Since steroids cause a loss of potassium, a diet rich in potassium is helpful. Citrus fruits and their juices, as well as bananas are helpful in increasing potassium intake. Patients with mild diabetes or a tendency to high blood sugar should restrict their diets when they are placed on steroids. These patients must have their blood sugars monitored and may require treatment such as oral hypoglycemic agents or insulin.

Steroids should always be taken with food to minimize stomach irritation. Patients with histories of stomach ulcers are best placed on a regimen of antiulcer medication while they are receiving corticosteroids.

Steroids weaken bones by interfering with the absorption of calcium from food. When calcium levels fall, calcium must be mobilized from the bone to return blood levels to normal, thereby reducing bone mass (osteoporosis). Corticosteroids also activate cells, called osteoclasts, which break down bone and inhibit bone-forming cells, called osteoblasts. The result is bone breakdown and an increased risk of fractures. Bone is constantly being broken down and rebuilt. With age, more bone is broken down than is replaced. Corticosteroids increase bone loss, regardless of age. Patients receiving corticosteroids should consume at least 1,500 milligrams of calcium and 800 international units of vitamin D a day, either through diet or supplements. Estrogen is recommended for women at or near menopause. A bone-density measurement is recommended for anyone starting a long course of corticosteroids.

Cromolyn Sodium

As noted, cromolyn sodium, a derivative of khellin, an Egyptian herbal remedy, is a useful anti-inflammatory agent that may be used as an alternative to inhaled corticosteroids. In severe patients, cromolyn sodium (Intal) may be used in conjunction with steroids. Since its introduction, cromolyn has been the anti-inflammatory drug of choice for childhood asthmatics. It is also the preferred anti-inflammatory agent during pregnancy. Like the inhaled corticosteroids, cromolyn is slow acting and therefore requires a trial of three to six weeks to assess response.

It is not clear how cromolyn sodium reduces inflammation. Some evidence has pointed to an action on allergy cells that prevents release of irritating chemicals which cause inflammation. There may also be an antagonistic action on nervous stimulation that prevents bronchoconstriction and reflex cough. Cromolyn sodium has also been useful in preventing exercise-induced asthma.

Cromolyn is available as an aerosol for metered-dose inhalers and in solution for nebulization. The recommended dosage is two puffs four times a day from an MDI or 20 milligrams in solution via a nebulizer, also four times a day.

Adverse Effects of Cromolyn

In addition to being an effective drug, cromolyn has a low incidence of side effects, which explains its first-line use in children where high-dose inhaled corticosteroids have been shown to slow bone development. In adults, the inhaled corticosteroids are considered more effective, making cromolyn a second-line agent. There are few adverse effects. Occasionally, cough and wheezing may result from its inhalation. This can often be prevented with the use of a B-adrenergic agonist sprayed five to ten minutes before use or given in solution with cromolyn via nebulization. Total-body effects have rarely been noted. A small number of patients have joint pains and rash. These effects are resolved completely on discontinuation.

Nedocromil Sodium

Nedocromil sodium (Tilade) resembles cromolyn sodium in its effects as an anti-inflammatory. Nedocromil, however, is structurally different from cromolyn and may also prevent the release of irritating chemicals that perpetuate the asthmatic reaction, but its mechanism of action is unknown.

Nedocromil is available as an aerosol delivered by metered-dose inhaler. Compared with cromolyn sodium, nedocromil appears to be more potent, and in large series of patients has been shown to be slightly more effective. The daily dosage is two puffs four times a day, but in stable patients it may be reduced to twice a day. Nedocromil should be regarded as an alternative to inhaled corticosteroids and cromolyn as a preventive anti-inflammatory. It may be particularly useful in cough asthma. Nedocromil has a slow onset of action and should be given three to six weeks before judgment of its effectiveness is made.

Adverse Effects of Nedocromil

Like cromolyn sodium, nedocromil has few total-body side effects. Patient acceptance, however, has been affected by a greater incidence of nausea after its use, as well as aftertaste and, occasionally, throat irritation. A flushing sensation can be noted after its use.

Leukotriene Antagonists/Inhibitors

An exciting addition to the anti-inflammatory drugs is a group of medications that affects the action and production of leukotrienes. Leukotrienes are produced when the walls of allergy cells break down as part of the allergic reaction. These irritating chemicals are one of several mediators of the inflammatory reaction. Numerous studies have demonstrated that this family of medications may reduce the frequency of asthmatic attacks. Patients receiving these agents are often able to reduce the use of both B_2-agonists and corticosteroids.

Zafirlukast

Zafirlukast (Accolate) acts as an antagonist by binding to receptor sites and blocking the action of one of the leukotrienes. It is taken orally, which offers an alternative for patients who do not tolerate aerosol sprays. The dosage of Zafirlukast is 20 milligrams twice a day taken an hour before or two hours after a meal. Zafirlukast may produce beneficial effects in days but requires at least a two-week period to determine a response to treatment.

Adverse Effects. Zafirlukast is usually well tolerated. Headache and nausea have been noted infrequently and rarely precipitate discontinuation of the drug. Six out of the first 270,000 Americans who took Zafirlukast were reported to have developed the Churg-Strauss syndrome, a rare disorder of small blood vessels (vasculitis). There is no evidence that Zafirlukast produced the syndrome in the six patients; rather, it may

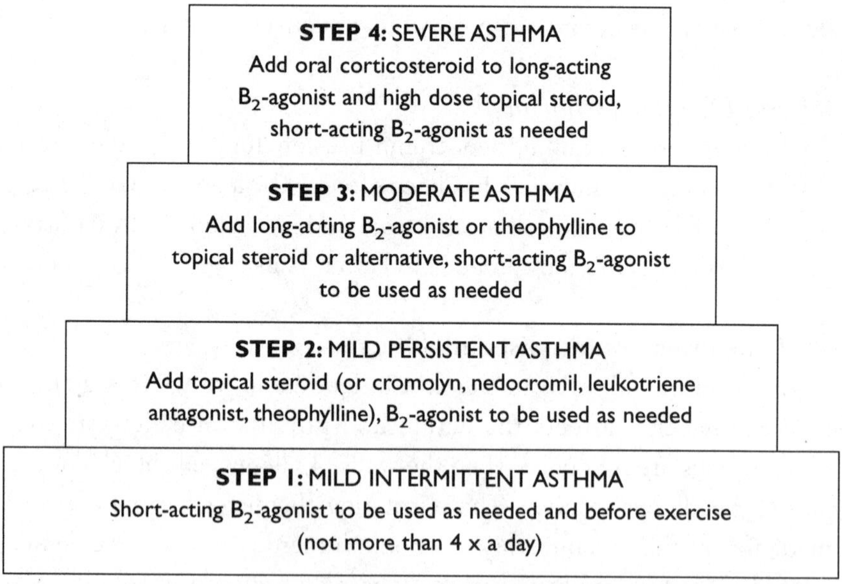

STEP 4: SEVERE ASTHMA
Add oral corticosteroid to long-acting
B₂-agonist and high dose topical steroid,
short-acting B₂-agonist as needed

STEP 3: MODERATE ASTHMA
Add long-acting B₂-agonist or theophylline to
topical steroid or alternative, short-acting B₂-agonist
to be used as needed

STEP 2: MILD PERSISTENT ASTHMA
Add topical steroid (or cromolyn, nedocromil, leukotriene
antagonist, theophylline), B₂-agonist to be used as needed

STEP 1: MILD INTERMITTENT ASTHMA
Short-acting B₂-agonist to be used as needed and before exercise
(not more than 4 x a day)

FIG. 3.3 STEPWISE APPROACH TO THE TREATMENT OF ASTHMA.

have occurred when corticosteroid dosage was reduced. Physicians are advised to reduce oral corticosteroids carefully in previously steroid-dependent asthmatics.

Zileuton

Zileuton (Zyflo) is a medication that acts by inhibiting the enzyme involved in the production of leukotrienes. The dosage of zileuton is 600 milligrams taken orally four times a day. It can be taken with food or on an empty stomach. After three months, the dosage may be reduced to 600 milligrams twice a day. A response to zileuton is usually noted in two weeks, with maximal effect achieved in one to four months.

Adverse Effects of Zileuton. Approximately 4 percent of patients taking zileuton will develop abnormal liver-function tests. Patients taking this medication should have their blood tests monitored on a monthly basis for the first few months after the start of this medication.

Strategy for the Treatment of Asthma

A stepwise approach to treatment (see Fig. 3.3) is used to gain and maintain control of asthma. This step therapy ensures that medication will be given in the proper dosage and that unnecessary medication will not be given. In general, therapy is initiated at a higher level at the onset of treatment to establish prompt control and is then "stepped down" to reduce the risk of adverse effects of medication.

Goals of Treatment

Treatment goals for asthma are maintaining a normal lifestyle, including vigorous exercise; reversing bronchial narrowing, inflammation, and irritability, thereby sustaining normal lung function; and avoiding adverse medication effects. Symptoms such as shortness of breath, wheezing, and coughing should be minimal. Hospitalization and emergency room visits should be prevented.

■ Asthma: Intermittent, Mild, Moderate, and Severe

To prescribe the correct asthma medication, the physician must grade patients according to the severity of their condition. The National Institutes of Health has categorized asthma as "mild intermittent," "mild persistent," "moderate persistent," and "severe persistent." Patients at any level may experience severe, life-threatening asthmatic attacks. These severe attacks may occur suddenly after long, symptom-free periods with normal lung function.

Mild Intermittent Asthma

Patients with mild intermittent asthma have symptoms two times a week or less frequently. Airflow measurements such as peak flow are more than 80 percent of normal. These patients do not require daily medication and use a short-acting B_2-agonist as needed for relief of symptoms.

Mild Persistent Asthma

Patients with mild persistent asthma have symptoms more than twice a week but less than once a day. Peak flow measurements are also more than 80 percent of normal. In these patients, the daily, regular use of an anti-inflammatory agent (low dose of inhaled corticosteroid, or cromolyn or nedocromil) is needed. The leukotriene antagonists/inhibitor and theophylline are considered alternative anti-inflammatory agents. For quick relief of symptoms, these patients will use a short-acting B_2-agonist.

Moderate Persistent Asthma

Patients with moderate persistent asthma have daily symptoms. Their peak flows are between 60 to 80 percent of normal. These patients require the addition of a long-acting B_2-agonist, such as salmeterol, to their daily regimen of an inhaled corticosteroid. Persistent nocturnal symptoms may also require the addition of theophylline. The leukotriene antagonists/inhibitor may also be helpful in this group. A short-acting B_2-agonist is used for quick relief.

Severe Persistent Asthma

Patients with severe persistent asthma have continuous symptoms and frequent asthmatic attacks. Peak flows are less than 60 percent of normal. These patients require high doses of inhaled corticosteroids, long-acting B_2-agonist, theophylline, and may require frequent or daily use of oral corticosteroids for control of symptoms. The short-acting B_2-agonist is used for quick relief of symptoms.

Physician-Patient Partnership

Treatment strategy must be developed by close communication (aided by peak flow measurements) between the patient and physician. Every asthmatic should have a written treatment plan that clearly indicates how medication should be administered.

CHRONIC OBSTRUCTIVE PULMONARY DISEASE (COPD)

Chronic obstructive pulmonary disease (COPD) is the fourth leading—and increasing—cause of death in the United States. In 1987, COPD was responsible for 74,000 deaths in the United States. In the same year, it prompted 11.2 million physician visits and 354,000 hospitalizations. The death rate has risen steadily, reaching 96,141 in 1994, with estimates of more than 100,000 casualties of this disease in 1996.

What Is COPD?

Chronic obstructive pulmonary disease is characterized by abnormal expiratory airflows over a prolonged period. It includes two major breathing disorders: emphysema and chronic bronchitis. Unlike asthma, COPD is not reversible.

Chronic obstructive pulmonary disease is primarily a disease of the middle-aged and elderly, which peaks between sixty-five and seventy-four years of age. Between fifty-five and sixty-four years of age it is more common in women. Of note, since 1980 the rate of COPD in men has been decreasing, while it has increased in women. This divergence has been largely attributed to changes in smoking habits. Each year, COPD–attributable deaths in the United States result in more than half a million years of potential life lost before the age of sixty-five. This statistic suggests that COPD not only attacks the elderly but is also a killer of individuals during their highly productive middle years.

A Smoker's Disease

Cigarettes have their most devastating impact on the respiratory system by causing COPD. The strong relationship between smoking and COPD has been recognized since the 1950s. In 1988, 61,660 people in the United States died of smoking-attributable COPD. For these individuals, death is usually preceded by a long period of suffering and disability. Approximately 16 million people, or 6 percent of the U.S. population, were estimated to be suffering from COPD in 1994. These patients required 743,089 hospitalizations per year.

Cigarette smoking produces three types of lung injuries—overproduction of mucus (causing cough and sputum production); airway narrowing with reduced expiratory airflows; and destruction of the walls of the alveolar air sacs. Abnormal lung-function tests are noted in the majority of long-term smokers, but only 15 percent will develop significant COPD. The fact that significant COPD does not develop in every cigarette smoker indicates that other factors, such as heredity and environment, are also involved.

Cigarette-induced lung damage begins in the small bronchial tubes and progresses to involve larger airways and the alveolar sacs. In the airways, increased numbers of white blood cells produce inflammation that results in increased mucus and narrowed passageways. It is thought that tobacco smoke destroys the air sacs by inhibiting an important enzyme, antiprotease. When antiprotease is prevented from acting, digestive enzymes, called proteases, are unchecked and digest the walls of the alveoli.

The lung damage produced by cigarette smoking becomes apparent with the development of shortness of breath and cough. This is a slow process that occurs over many years. It is not clear if exposure to smoke as a child predisposes the adult to the development of COPD.

Other Factors Causing COPD

Cigarette smoking also produces lung damage by affecting the lung's natural defense mechanisms. Smokers mount a weakened immune response to organisms that produce respiratory infection. Smoking also impacts the sweeping action of the delicate projections (cilia) on the lining surface of the bronchial tubes; thus, cigarette smokers have more frequent respiratory infections. These infections may predispose the patient to the development of COPD. Several studies have also implicated viral infections at an early age in the development of COPD.

Air pollution due to the burning of coal has been known to produce chronic bronchitis in the United States and Great Britain, but efforts aimed at reducing this pollution have had a substantial effect. Exposure to other pollutants, such as sulfur dioxide, nitrogen dioxide, and particulates, leads to a decline in lung function. During days with high pollution levels, emergency room admissions for exacerbations of COPD increase significantly.

Heredity is also thought to play a significant role in the development of COPD. Individuals who are deficient in an enzyme, alpha$_1$-antitrypsin (AAT), are known to develop emphysema at an early age, often in their thirties or forties. Individuals with chronic bronchitis are twice as likely to have a family history of the disease. Abnormalities in pulmonary function tests are common in parents and siblings of patients with COPD.

Allergy may also play a role. Numerous patients with COPD are allergic and have elevated levels of IgE. The bronchial tubes in COPD tend to be hyperresponsive, a feature that is common in allergy. This hyperresponsiveness may predispose the air tubes to constrict when exposed to tobacco smoke, infection, or other lung irritants.

Chronic Bronchitis

Chronic bronchitis is defined by the presence of a mucous-producing cough most days of the month, three months of the year, for two successive years without other underlying disease to explain the cough. This breathing disorder may precede or accompany emphysema. It is unusual to find an individual with chronic bronchitis who does not also have some component of emphysema, and vice versa. It is estimated that 5 percent of the population is affected by chronic bronchitis. In 1993, approximately 13.8 million people suffered from this disease. It ranked sixth in prevalence among all chronic conditions and was responsible for 878,000 physician visits in 1992.

In bronchitis, the delicate lining (mucosa) of the airways is inflamed. The mucous-secreting glands within the walls of the bronchial tubes respond to irritation by producing excessive amounts of thick mucus. This secretion and the inflamed, swollen passageways obstruct the flow of air through the bronchial tubes.

Acute bronchitis is a common illness in which infection produces a chest cold characterized by cough and sputum production.

CAUSES OF CHRONIC BRONCHITIS

Chronic bronchitis is a disease of cigarette smokers, which begins when tobacco smoke produces irritation of the bronchial tubes. Bacterial and viral infections frequently play a role in the development of this disease. Once the bronchial tubes become inflamed and clogged with mucus, repeated bouts of acute infection are common.

In many cases, air pollution and industrial dusts are also causative factors. Higher rates of bronchitis are found among coal miners, grain handlers, metal molders, and other workers exposed to dust. This may be called "industrial bronchitis."

SYMPTOMS OF CHRONIC BRONCHITIS

The most common symptom of chronic bronchitis is a productive cough with expectoration of phlegm. Patients frequently describe having a winter chest cold that continues to produce cough and large amounts of discolored mucus for several weeks. Since many of these individuals are cigarette smokers, the cough is often dismissed as a smoker's cough.

Episodes of repeated infection with increased cough and phlegm last longer and longer after each chest cold, until the cough becomes continuous, year-round. Patients describe a pattern of severe coughing on arising in the morning, with production of yellow or green sputum.

The cough of a patient with chronic bronchitis is distinctive. My consultation room is adjacent to the office's waiting room so I often hear a variety of coughs. In many instances, I feel that I can make a diagnosis even before I actually see a patient by first hearing her cough. Patients with chronic bronchitis have a loud, deep-seated, and phlegmy cough. The patient experiences severe paroxysms of coughing that may last several minutes.

In 75 percent of patients with chronic bronchitis, cough precedes the onset of shortness of breath, or the two symptoms occur simultaneously.

SIGNS OF CHRONIC BRONCHITIS:
THE "BLUE BLOATER"

Patients with chronic bronchitis may have characteristic physical findings. Due to a high incidence of cyanosis and heart failure in severe cases, these patients have been called "blue bloaters." On physical examination, a bluish skin discoloration, cyanosis, which is due to a low

oxygen level, may be noticeable. Elevation of carbon dioxide may produce somnolence. The abnormal blood gases may lead to heart failure
and swelling of the legs.

The chest examination is remarkable for a number of musical sounds.
As air passes through the mucous-clogged airways, turbulence is produced.
The turbulent airflow typically produces wheezes that are high pitched,
and rhonchi, which are of a lower pitch. This "symphony" of sounds may
be altered suddenly by cough and the expectoration of mucus.

LABORATORY FINDINGS IN CHRONIC BRONCHITIS

The diagnosis of chronic bronchitis is based on the patient's history of
cough over a period of time. No single laboratory finding can be used to
make this diagnosis.

Chest x-rays of patients with chronic bronchitis may reveal promi-
nence of the bronchial markings. This so-called "dirty chest" is often seen
in cigarette smokers as well. In patients with low oxygen and high carbon
dioxide levels, there may be enlargement of the right side of the heart.

Pulmonary function tests in patients with chronic bronchitis are
often helpful in supporting the diagnosis. Via spirometry, we see varying
degrees of airway obstruction. This may be characterized as mild, moderate, or severe when compared with normal standards.

Emphysema

In emphysema, the thin walls of the alveoli break down, forming larger
air pockets in the lungs and producing a loss of elasticity. Normal lungs
contain a substance called elastin, which gives cells in the air sacs the
ability to snap back and exhale air after it is inhaled. When the lungs are
exposed to the irritation of cigarette smoke, the body responds by send-
ing immune cells, called macrophages, to the site of irritation. These
cells produce an enzyme, called elastase, which destroys the air sacs,
resulting in emphysema.

The loss of elasticity due to emphysema makes it difficult to exhale, trapping air in damaged spaces of the lung. This trapped air produces overinflation, which further interferes with the normal exchange of oxygen and carbon dioxide.

CAUSES OF EMPHYSEMA

As discussed, cigarette smoking is the primary cause of emphysema. It has been estimated that smoking is responsible for 82 percent of chronic lung disease. Air pollution and occupational exposures to irritating fumes and dust are also suspected causes.

A deficiency of the enzyme $alpha_1$-antitrypsin (AAT) is a rare hereditary form of emphysema that affects an estimated 50,000 to 100,000 Americans. These patients lack this protective protein that normally prevents digestion of the walls of the air sacs by destructive (proteolytic) enzymes.

SYMPTOMS OF EMPHYSEMA

Shortness of breath is the most frequent symptom of emphysema. These patients often have severe air hunger. The course of emphysema is slow and gradual, initially producing breathlessness with exercise. As the disease progresses, patients may notice shortness of breath with walking and more routine activities. Unfortunately, most patients do not consult their physicians until symptoms worsen. A common precipitating reason for consultation is the development of an upper respiratory tract infection, which increases breathlessness.

As noted above, chronic bronchitis often accompanies emphysema so that patients may also present with cough and sputum production.

Weight loss is also seen frequently in patients with severe disease. At times, weight loss may be profound and suggest underlying malignancy. The cause of this weight loss is not clear but is most likely due to an increase in energy expenditure or "work of breathing." This increased work results from the increased use of calories by the breathing muscles such as the diaphragm. This increased consumption may be compounded by poor nutrition.

Psychiatric disturbances such as anxiety and depression occur frequently. COPD patients and especially those with emphysema are often victims of hopelessness resulting from an inability to carry out normal activities. Sleep disturbances and loss of memory may also be present and may be due to low oxygen levels.

SIGNS OF EMPHYSEMA: THE "PINK PUFFER"

Patients with emphysema take rapid, shallow breaths and experience great difficulty exhaling. The rapid breathing pattern often compensates for drops in oxygen levels so that these patients are pink and not blue. For many years, the term "pink puffer" has been used to describe their appearance.

The increased work of breathing of these patients is often demonstrated by the use of the muscles of the neck with each breath. The overinflation of the lung may increase the width of the chest ("barrel-chested") and lower the position of the diaphragm.

Breath sounds are typically diminished in intensity so that the physician may find the patient's chest sounds to be nearly absent in patients with severe disease. The loss of elasticity in emphysema also produces early closing of air passages. The resulting turbulent airflow may produce wheezing.

It should be stressed that there is considerable overlap between patients with emphysema and chronic bronchitis so that many patients have a combination of the two disorders.

LABORATORY FINDINGS IN EMPHYSEMA

Although only a small number of patients has the rare inherited form of emphysema called alpha$_1$-antitrypsin deficiency, blood testing for this enzyme deficiency should be performed in all patients with COPD.

Overinflation of the lungs is frequently noted by chest x-ray in patients with emphysema. (See Fig. 3.4.) This finding, however, is not specific for this disorder because it may also occur in asthma. Large air-containing, cystlike areas (bullae) are often noted in advanced cases of emphysema. However, bullae may also be present from birth. CAT scanning has been increasingly used in the evaluation of patients with

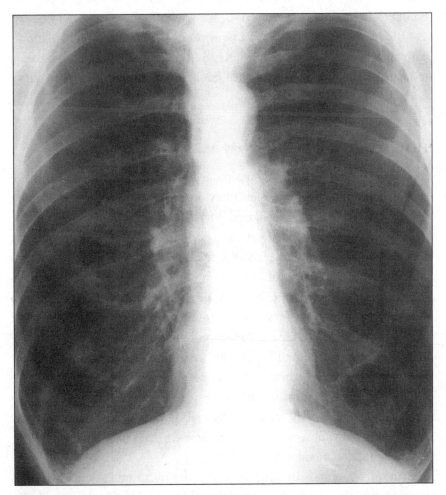

FIG. 3.4 CHEST X-RAY IN EMPHYSEMA (the lungs appear larger and darker than normal).

emphysema because it can detect destruction of air sacs sooner than a plain chest x-ray can. It may also be used before lung-reduction surgery.

Pulmonary function tests are helpful in diagnosing emphysema. The loss of elasticity in emphysema produces varying degrees of obstruction to airflow. Partial reversibility may be seen after the use of a bronchodilator. Lung volumes often document the overinflation of the lung. The diffusion capacity is characteristically reduced due to the destruction of the alveoli.

Blood oxygen levels may not be severely decreased in many patients with mild to moderate emphysema. As the disease progresses, oxygen levels usually decrease significantly, and carbon dioxide levels rise above normal.

HOW COPD DIFFERS FROM ASTHMA

Asthma and COPD share many similar features, such as narrowed, congested, and inflamed bronchial tubes. One major difference is that the breathing function of asthmatics fluctuates a great deal, whereas the COPD patient usually has relatively fixed lung function and unchanging symptoms. (See Table 3.6.) Another feature of patients with COPD is a gradual decline in lung function with aging, such that these patients may become incapacitated by their disease. This is especially true in patients who continue to smoke. The asthmatic patient, on the other hand, usually does not have progressive loss of breathing function.

Spirometry performed before and after the use of a bronchodilator may also distinguish asthma from chronic bronchitis. Asthma is, by definition, a reversible form of airway obstruction so that after the bronchodilator, airflows may return to normal. Patients with COPD usually have fixed airflow obstruction or may demonstrate only partial reversibility after the bronchodilator.

Another useful distinguishing test is the diffusion capacity, which is usually normal in asthmatics but reduced in COPD patients.

Patients with severe COPD demonstrate marked abnormalities in blood gases—elevated carbon dioxide and lower oxygen levels. These changes are unusual in asthma except for severe asthmatic attacks, where they are reversed with aggressive treatment.

THE TREATMENT OF COPD

The treatment of COPD is directed at eliminating irritation in the air tubes, while providing appropriate medication. Improvement of "bronchial hygiene" is particularly important in chronic bronchitis patients who have excess secretion. A comprehensive treatment program also includes proper nutrition, frequent exercise, stress reduction, and weight reduction. In selected patients with emphysema, surgery may now be a viable option.

TABLE 3.6 COMPARING COPD AND ASTHMA

Feature	COPD	Asthma
Age	Older	Younger
Bronchial narrowing	Constant	Intermittent
Course after diagnosis	Tends to grow worse over time	Variable; usually favorable
Effect of bronchodilator	Mild	Marked; may be dramatic
Effect of exercise	Oxygen levels drop	Constricts airways
Pulmonary function tests	Low diffusion capacity; higher CO_2, response to bronchodilator mild	Normal diffusion capacity; low CO_2, marked response to bronchodilator

You Must Stop Smoking!

Among the many treatment options, the most important is smoking cessation. Numerous studies have demonstrated the benefits of quitting. Within one month of quitting, many patients report a dramatic decrease in cough, wheezing, shortness of breath, and the amount of sputum expectorated. This improvement may occur regardless of the number of years and packs per day that an individual has smoked.

Individuals who stop smoking have fewer respiratory infections than those who continue. This is especially important in COPD, where respiratory infections frequently exacerbate this disease.

Pulmonary function tests may also improve. Studies of airflows have demonstrated significant improvement in many patients six to twelve

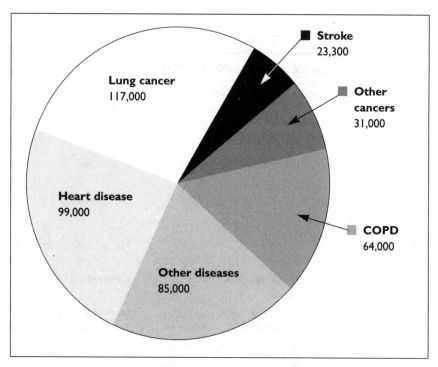

FIG. 3.5　THE DEATH TOLL FROM CIGARETTE SMOKING FOR 1990.

months after smoking cessation. In many patients with COPD, no longer smoking prevents further decline in lung function by arresting the production of additional damage. Those patients who continue to smoke have an accelerated deterioration in breathing function, usually manifested by increased shortness of breath. This can be avoided by not smoking.

About Staying Alive

Despite the fact that there has been a decline in the number of smokers in the last twenty-five years, the death rate resulting from cigarette smoking has steadily increased. This phenomenon occurs due to a lag period from the time of exposure to cigarette smoke to the onset of illness. This lag period is often ten to twenty years. The current death rate from cigarette smoking reflects the prevalence of smoking in the 1960s and 1970s.

As of 1990, approximately 419,000 deaths in the United States were directly attributable to cigarette smoking. (See Fig. 3.5.) It has been estimated that one out of every five deaths in this country can be directly attributed to cigarette smoking. In 1990, smoking resulted in nearly 117,000 deaths from lung cancer, 31,000 deaths from other cancers, 23,300 deaths from stroke, 64,000 deaths from COPD, 99,000 deaths from heart disease, and 85,000 deaths from other causes. Based on these data, cigarettes were responsible for the loss of more than five million years of potential life in 1990. This information makes the message clear—staying alive means not smoking.

How to Quit

It has been argued that the most effective way to eliminate lung disease in the United States would be to eliminate cigarette smoking. Although greater restrictions have been placed on cigarette smoking, the decline in smoking has been modest—perhaps because of the strong addictive nature of nicotine. With the proper support and guidance, however, anyone can stop smoking.

The decision to quit should start with a discussion with your physician about the damaging effects of smoking and the potential benefits of quitting. It is often helpful to review the results of pulmonary function tests to illustrate the effects of tobacco smoke on the lungs. Once the decision is made, a "quit date" is set. It is also helpful to sign and have witnessed a contract with the physician to quit smoking.

The physician can assess the degree of physical addiction as opposed to the psychological need for smoking. The physical craving may be reduced by using a nicotine substitute (gum, patch, nasal spray). The use of the nicotine patch during withdrawal has more than doubled the number of people who were able to quit smoking.

Many medications have also been used to decrease craving and may be prescribed by your physician. These include clonidine (Catapres), a medication that is normally prescribed for control of high blood pressure. This drug appears to have limited application due to its effect on blood pressure. Buspirone (Buspar), an anxiety-reducing medication, has also been shown to be helpful in smoking cessation.

Bupropion Hydrochloride (Zyban)

A low dose of an antidepressant medication, bupropion hydrochloride, Zyban, has recently been approved for smoking cessation and appears helpful. In a recent study of adult smokers, 23.1 percent of those receiving bupropion hydrochloride were still not smoking after one year compared with a success rate of 12.4 percent of patients who received a placebo. This medication also appears to significantly reduce the weight gain experienced by individuals who quit smoking. This weight gain is often a deterrent to many intended nonsmokers. In selected patients, bupropion hydrochloride may also be used in conjunction with a nicotine substitute.

Antibiotic Therapy in COPD

Antibiotic therapy may be helpful in treating exacerbations of COPD. Numerous studies of the effect of antibiotic on flare-ups of COPD have shown that this form of medication shortens the illness and reduces cough and shortness of breath. One study revealed that the use of antibiotics in this setting reduced by 50 percent the likelihood of hospitalization. Pulmonary function tests have also been shown to improve after the use of antibiotics.

This treatment is usually given by mouth over a period of ten to fourteen days. Whenever possible, a sputum sample should be obtained by the physician for culture. This simple procedure may isolate the infecting organism that has produced the flare-up of this condition. In addition to isolating the organism, the laboratory will routinely run a sensitivity test to determine which antibiotics will be most effective. Sputum cultures may not always yield a specific organism. In these instances, and when sputum is unavailable for culture, the physician must decide empirically on the specific antibiotic.

Bronchodilator Therapy

Bronchodilator therapy may be beneficial in relieving cough and shortness of breath in patients with COPD. Although the response to these agents is not as dramatic as that seen in asthma, significant reduction in symptoms has been well documented.

Ipratropium Bromide: Alone or in Combination

The preferred bronchodilator for patients with COPD is the anticholinergic agent ipratropium bromide (Atrovent). A significant improvement in airflows has also been seen with the use of the short-acting B_2-adrenergic agonists. When these two types of bronchodilators are combined, a greater effect than that seen with either agent alone has been demonstrated. A spray that combines albuterol sulfate with ipratropium bromide (Combivent) is now available.

The long-acting B_2-adrenergic agonist, salmeterol (Serevent), has been demonstrated to significantly reduce symptoms of patients with COPD. This agent may be helpful in patients in whom ipratropium bromide is contraindicated—those with closed angle glaucoma or enlarged prostate glands.

Theophylline should be considered a second-line bronchodilator for patients with COPD. Recent research has focused on a beneficial effect of theophylline on the strength of contraction of the diaphragm in these patients. Since the diaphragm is an overworked muscle in patients with COPD, this effect may reduce shortness of breath. However, the adverse effects of theophylline, especially in the elderly population, may outweigh any benefit.

Corticosteroids in COPD

The use of corticosteroids in the treatment of COPD has been the subject of much debate. It appears that steroids may be beneficial in a small number of patients. A recent study found that 11 percent of patients with COPD treated with oral corticosteroids showed significant improvement in pulmonary function. In many of these cases, the patients had asthmalike symptoms and features. These data illustrate that there is considerable overlap in many patients who have components of asthma, chronic bronchitis, and emphysema.

Inhaled corticosteroids do not appear to help most patients with COPD. In the patients who respond to oral steroids, however, the inhaled steroids sprays may prove beneficial.

Oxygen Therapy

The only treatment that has been shown to lengthen the life span of patients with COPD is the use of oxygen therapy. Oxygen therapy has also been shown to improve the quality of life and intelligence quotient of patients after six months of therapy. Patients treated with oxygen often report that they sleep better, have fewer nightmares, and awake with more energy.

Oxygen therapy is *only* beneficial in those COPD patients with severely reduced oxygen levels. Oxygen does little to relieve air hunger in many "pink puffers."

Whenever oxygen is used, the flow must be closely regulated. It is best to regard oxygen as a drug and to manage its administration as carefully as any medication. In selected patients, too much oxygen may indeed prove harmful—even fatal. This phenomenon relates to the control of breathing. In patients who have higher levels of carbon dioxide, the controlling neurons in the brain depend on input from the peripheral oxygen receptors to drive breathing. In these patients, high oxygen levels essentially turn off the vital receptor and further depress breathing.

How Oxygen Is Administered in the Home

Oxygen therapy may be administered in the home to patients with severe COPD. Three types of devices are commonly used: high-pressure oxygen cylinders, or tanks; liquid oxygen; and oxygen concentrators.

High-pressure oxygen cylinders are manufactured in various sizes. The large H cylinder is often used as a reservoir in the home, while the smaller E tank is commonly used when the patient goes out. The E tank can be pushed on a dolly and is light enough to be placed in a car. The drawback of tank oxygen is that once the cylinder gas is emptied, it must be replaced and refilled.

Liquid oxygen is used primarily as a portable unit because the canisters are lightweight and allow the patient to be more active. The portable units are filled from a larger home reservoir. Liquid oxygen is more expensive than cylinder O_2, and the home reservoirs must be filled frequently.

The oxygen concentrator has become the most common source of home O_2. This electrical device creates oxygen by drawing in room air and filtering it through a membrane so that oxygen is separated from nitrogen. Unlike tank and liquid oxygen, which deliver 100 percent O_2, the oxygen concentrator delivers 90 percent O_2. This discrepancy requires a slight adjustment in the amount of oxygen administered. Patients with oxygen concentrators require a backup unit, usually an E or H cylinder, in case of a power failure.

How Much Oxygen Should Be Given?

The amount or flow of oxygen is determined by the physician from the patient's blood level. As noted, too much oxygen can be dangerous and the amount is always individualized.

The COPD patient, however, typically requires "low flow" oxygen (expressed as liters per minute), which is delivered through plastic tubing. A commonly used device is a nasal cannula, which sits just below the nose with two short extensions (prongs) that enter the nostrils. Oxygen is delivered despite the fact that the patient may breathe through the mouth. In selected patients, a face mask may be more effective and may be substituted for the nasal cannula.

Lung-Reduction Surgery
In many patients with COPD, the lungs contain large air-filled spaces, which are formed when the walls of the small alveoli break down. Some of these cystlike structures may be quite large. One of the effects of the enlarged air spaces is to produce overexpansion of the lung, which in turn pushes down on the diaphragm.

Lung-reduction surgery has been recently used in selected COPD patients to relieve symptoms, particularly shortness of breath. Several different surgical approaches have been used, including video-guided techniques. One series of more than two hundred patients reported significant improvement in the majority of patients for the first year after lung reduction.

Pulmonary function tests in the patients undergoing surgery reveal improvement in airflows and reduction in hyperinflation. Postoperative chest x-rays often reveal elevation of the diaphragm to its normal position.

Lung reduction is not without risk, however, and remains controversial. The cost of this procedure is not yet reimbursable under Medicare. In 1995, the National Institutes of Health began a seven-year nationwide study of lung-reduction surgery in COPD, called the National Emphysema Treatment Trial, or NETT, comparing the results of surgery with pulmonary rehabilitation. The NIH hopes to enroll 2,600 patients in this nationwide study.

Lung Transplantation
Lung transplantation continues to make strides toward greater success rates but remains an option for only a small number of patients.

The Future: Stimulating the Immune System
Patients with COPD often suffer deterioration after repeated bouts of respiratory tract infection. One future treatment for this condition is aimed at stimulating the immune system to protect against these infections.

Preliminary results of the use of an oral vaccine, called Pseudostat, in patients with chronic bronchitis are encouraging. This vaccine stimulates the production of protective white blood cells, which neutralize invading bacteria. A recent study of COPD patients receiving Pseudostat found a marked reduction in the number of respiratory infections.

Treatment for AAT Deficiency–Related Emphysema

Alpha$_1$-Protease Inhibitor
In patients with AAT deficiency–related emphysema, treatment with alpha$_1$-protease inhibitor (Prolastin) restores the blood level of this enzyme to normal. This treatment is given once a week by intravenous infusion and is safe and well tolerated. These patients must have documented AAT deficiency and airflow obstruction. The long-term benefits of this treatment are not known.

The Future: Gene Therapy for AAT Deficiency
Research has pinpointed the specific problem in AAT deficiency. A single gene, located on chromosome number 14, bears the code that triggers the production of AAT in the liver. Patients with AAT deficiency who are missing this gene may one day be treated by delivering to the liver DNA carrying the code.

Pulmonary Rehabilitation
Pulmonary rehabilitation involves the use of several disciplines, with the goal of improving the functional state of COPD patients. Its primary goal is to improve the patient's quality of life. For the majority of sufferers, pulmonary rehabilitation aims at restoring the ability to function without extreme breathing distress. This is accomplished through

graduated exercise programs, usually incorporating the use of a tread-mill. Additional exercises to strengthen the upper body and breathing muscles are also utilized. Although pulmonary function does not improve with rehabilitation, exercise tolerance does. This often allows the patient to eat, shower, dress, and leave the home for normal daily activities without experiencing severe shortness of breath.

A comprehensive rehabilitation program should also address the patient's nutritional and psychological needs. The needs of family members must also be addressed. (Specific features of pulmonary rehabilitation are discussed in Chapter 7.)

Treating Anxiety and Depression

Patients with COPD often require treatment of anxiety and depression. This is best done in consultation with a psychiatrist or psychologist. Counseling and biofeedback may be helpful in selected patients. Anti-depressant and anxiety-reducing medication may also be necessary. In considering medication, the physician must avoid drugs that are known to depress breathing. As a general rule, tranquilizers and sleeping pills should be avoided in patients with COPD.

Don't Forget Influenza and Pneumonia Vaccines

The prevention of respiratory infection may be lifesaving in patients with COPD. Influenza and pneumonia may produce severe illness in these patients, often requiring hospitalization. Influenza vaccine is given on a yearly basis. A vaccine against the most common form of pneumococcal, bacterial pneumonia, has been available since 1977. In 1983, Pneumovax was reformulated to include several more strains of this bacteria. It is recommended that anyone who received the older formula should be revaccinated with the newer vaccine. The protection afforded by this vaccine has been shown to last five to ten years in most patients. Those individuals who are judged to be at high risk for pneumonia may be revaccinated after five years.

Watch Out for Beta-Blockers

Beta-blockers are commonly prescribed medications for high blood pressure and heart disease. They are often used to control irregular heart rhythms, as well as in the patient with coronary artery disease. In addition, beta-blockers have been used in the treatment of migraines, tremors, and glaucoma (as an eyedrop). These popular medications, however, may have adverse effects in patients with asthma and COPD.

When active or stimulated, the beta-receptors in the lung (called beta-2 receptors) produce relaxation of the muscle surrounding the bronchial tubes, which widens the bronchial passage (bronchodilatation). If these receptors are blocked from receiving nerve input, the reverse effect (bronchoconstriction) may result. This may have devastating effects on patients with asthma and COPD. Patients who are given these medications (including eyedrop preparations) may notice wheezing or increased shortness of breath.

Beta-receptors are present in other organ systems, including the heart and circulation, and are referred to as beta-1 receptors. Beta-blocker medications that affect beta-1 receptors more than beta-2 receptors are termed "selective." These medications vary in potency and duration. Several selective beta-blockers produce less blockage of lung receptors, but there still is a risk of exacerbating COPD and asthma. Whenever possible, beta-blockers should be avoided in patients with COPD and asthma.

BRONCHIECTASIS

Bronchiectasis, a disease of the lung's airways, indicates that the wall of the bronchial tube is permanently damaged. This damage usually results from untreated bronchial infection. The damage means a widening or dilatation of the bronchial tube. This dilatation may take several forms. One of the most common is the formation of many sacs or pouches in the wall of the air tubes. These warm, moist, dark spaces are a breeding ground for bacteria that produce recurrent infection.

Causes of Bronchiectasis

The most common cause of bronchiectasis, a severe infection of the lower respiratory tract, damages the bronchial tubes. This infection may be viral, such as influenza, or bacterial and may take the form of bronchitis or pneumonia. In some cases, bronchiectasis is produced by repeated episodes of infection. Many elderly patients developed bronchiectasis due to whooping cough (pertussis) or tuberculosis prior to the development of effective treatment or vaccination. Individuals with cystic fibrosis—abnormal mucus obstructs the bronchial tubes—characteristically develop severe bronchiectasis.

Bronchiectasis may also be produced by noninfectious causes. One of the most common is the aspiration of stomach contents into the lungs. This material contains stomach acid and food particles, which irritate and damage the bronchial tubes. Aspiration may occur under many circumstances. It occurs frequently with drug overdoses, when the normal protective reflexes that prevent aspiration are depressed.

A common condition known as gastroesophageal reflux may also cause aspiration and lead to bronchiectasis. In this disorder, the muscle sphincter, which closes the end of the feeding tube (esophagus) as it connects to the stomach, malfunctions, allowing a backward movement of stomach contents.

Foreign bodies may be accidentally inhaled into the bronchial tubes and produce inflammation. If these objects are not detected and removed, the inflammation may progress to infection and bronchiectasis.

Symptoms of Bronchiectasis

The most striking feature of bronchiectasis is a persistent cough productive of large amounts of discolored sputum. The sputum is often thick and may be putrid. Patients with bronchiectasis frequently experience blood-spitting, or hemoptysis. In severe cases, shortness of breath, fatigue, and weight loss are common.

Signs of Bronchiectasis

Patients with bronchiectasis have abnormal chest sounds due to the presence of large amounts of mucus in the bronchial tubes. Low-pitched, rumbling sounds and wheezes are common. Patients frequently expectorate during the examination. In severe cases, cyanosis may be present, as well as a curvature of the nails, called clubbing. Sinusitis is frequently found in patients with bronchiectasis.

How Is Bronchiectasis Diagnosed?

The most useful method of diagnosis is the chest CAT scan, which reveals the ballooning or dilatation of the bronchial tubes. A chest x-ray may also indicate bronchiectasis. Prior to the development of the CAT scanner, a technique known as bronchography, whereby dye was injected into the bronchial tubes, was used for diagnosis. Today, this procedure is rarely done.

Treatment of Bronchiectasis

ANTIBIOTICS

Antibiotics may be helpful in the management of bronchiectasis. Treatment is usually started when there is an exacerbation that produces shortness of breath, blood-spitting, fever, or increased cough and sputum production. Some patients may benefit from continuous or regular administration of antibiotics but run the risk of developing drug resistance.

CHEST PHYSIOTHERAPY

Chest physiotherapy is a time-honored procedure that utilizes gravity to promote drainage of thick mucus from the damaged bronchial tubes. This simple technique reduces the opportunity for bacteria to cause recurrent infection. During chest physiotherapy, the patient assumes various positions (postural drainage) while an assistant claps the back to help dislodge secretions. To avoid trauma, the clapping must be performed in a correct manner.

This procedure should be performed on waking and again, before sleep. With proper instruction from a chest physiotherapist, the patient's spouse can provide clapping. Electric vibrating devices may also be used to help loosen mucus.

TREAT THE UNDERLYING CONDITION

When bronchiectasis results from another condition, such as sinusitis, it is essential to correct the contributing disorder.

Sinusitis is often associated with bronchiectasis. Antibiotics may be necessary here as well to eradicate infection that drains into the airways. Sinus drainage may be facilitated by the use of anti-inflammatory sprays that shrink swollen mucous membranes.

Gastroesophageal reflux can be treated by elevating the head of one's bed and by not eating for two hours before bedtime. Alcohol and caffeine should also be avoided. Several medications are available for the treatment of reflux, including antacids, as well as drugs that reduce acid production and tighten the sphincter muscle.

IS SURGERY NECESSARY?

In patients with bronchiectasis localized to one portion of the lung, surgery is another treatment option. Before considering surgery, a chest CAT scan must be done to determine if multiple areas of the lung are damaged. If only one segment or lobe is found to be involved, pulmonary function tests are performed to determine if there is adequate reserve to permit removal of the lung. It is also important to evaluate the patient's general health and nutritional status prior to considering surgery.

CYSTIC FIBROSIS (CF)

Cystic fibrosis is an inherited lung disease that occurs once in every 3,500 births. It occurs more often in white children (once in 2,500 births) than in other racial groups. It is this country's most common fatal genetic defect. There are more than thirty thousand patients with CF in the United States and 55,000 worldwide. Life expectancy averages twenty-nine years. Advances in treatment, however, have increased survival of individual patients into their thirties and forties.

The specific gene responsible for CF was discovered in 1989. Since that time, scientists have discovered several hundred abnormalities or mutations in this gene. Due to these varied abnormalities, the severity of CF may vary from person to person. Some cases are mild, so the disease may not be detected in childhood. These adult patients have often been misdiagnosed as having chronic bronchitis or bronchiectasis.

What Causes CF?

Cystic fibrosis occurs when a gene located on chromosome number 7 fails to make its normal protein product. This protein functions as a duct in the outer membrane of cells through which chemicals pass. Two of these chemicals are sodium and chloride. The affected cells, called epithelial cells, line the surface passages of many organs, including the lungs and pancreas. As a result of the CF defect, the amount of sodium and chloride increases within the cells, drawing water from the lung's airways.

AN ABNORMAL MUCUS

In CF, the body produces an abnormally thick, sticky, dehydrated mucus. In the bronchial tubes, this viscous material clogs the air passages, trapping bacteria that produce recurrent infections (pneumonia, bronchitis). The result is bronchiectasis and destruction of alveoli by chemicals released by the bacteria.

The effects of CF are most evident in the lungs. Respiratory complications account for 90 percent of the deaths attributed to this disease. However, other organs are also affected by the abnormal mucus. In the pancreas, for example, obstruction of normal channels prevents enzymes from reaching the intestines, preventing one from digesting food.

How Is CF Inherited?

The cystic fibrosis gene is recessive, meaning that an individual must inherit two copies—one from each parent—in order to be affected. Approximately 5 percent of Americans of European descent (one in twenty) are believed to carry the defective gene.

Symptoms of Cystic Fibrosis

CF symptoms are primarily due to the recurrent chest infections that begin in infancy. In the older child, a persistent cough that is productive of sputum or shortness of breath may prompt a medical evaluation. The sputum is often discolored and may be blood streaked. As repeated infections occur, wheezing and shortness of breath may be noted. In some patients, nasal polyps and sinus infections are frequent, leading to complaints of blockage of the nasal passages, headache, and nasal discharge.

SYMPTOMS FROM OUTSIDE THE CHEST

In many CF patients, symptoms may occur as a result of involvement of other organs. Individuals with CF may develop bowel obstruction or liver disease. The blockage of the pancreas may result in abdominal pain, diarrhea, and malnutrition.

Infertility May Suggest Cystic Fibrosis

Ninety percent of men with cystic fibrosis are infertile as a result of a genetic defect called congenital absence of the vas deferens. The vas deferens are small ducts that carry sperm from the testicles to the penis. In patients with mild forms of CF, infertility may be the initial complaint that brings the individual to the physician.

Signs of Cystic Fibrosis

In most patients, the physical findings reflect repeated chest infections. In more severe cases, weight loss and cyanosis may be noted. Wheezing and rhonchi are usually present on examination of the chest. Patients with severe disease may have signs of heart failure, such as leg swelling or an enlarged liver.

How Is Cystic Fibrosis Diagnosed?

THE SWEAT TEST

Patients with cystic fibrosis have saltier-than-normal sweat due to the defect in cell membranes. This characteristic of more than 98 percent of patients with CF forms the basis of the sweat test, which is used for diagnosis. In this simple but useful test, the patient's arm is placed under a heat lamp. Sweat is collected after several minutes and analyzed for the amount of chloride.

The finding of an increased sweat chloride combined with the presence of chronic pulmonary or pancreatic disease currently forms the basis for the diagnosis of cystic fibrosis. Genetic testing (DNA analysis), however, is soon likely to replace the sweat test.

DNA TESTING

DNA testing can detect 70 to 75 percent of carriers of the defective gene that causes CF. This percentage is expected to increase as more mutations of the CF gene are identified. Scientists expect to identify more than three hundred mutations of this gene.

The most common mutation, called D508, causes about 68 percent of all cystic fibrosis cases. Most of the other mutations are rare and cause few cases of cystic fibrosis. Recently, a mutation called R117H has been found to be more common than was believed. It appears to sometimes cause cystic fibrosis, male sterility, chronic bronchitis, and sinusitis.

A reliable screening test for newborns, as well as prenatal screening, are available.

THE CHEST X-RAY IN CYSTIC FIBROSIS

Patients with cystic fibrosis have characteristic x-ray findings. These include bronchiectasis, fibrosis, cyst formation, and swollen lymph glands. Although these findings are typical of CF, they may also be seen in patients with other chest diseases, such as tuberculosis and sarcoidosis.

RESULTS OF SPUTUM CULTURE

Analysis of the sputum of patients with cystic fibrosis may be helpful in the treatment of this disease. Certain bacteria, such as *pseudomonas aeruginosa*, are frequently recovered in laboratory cultures. However, the presence of this and other bacteria is not sufficient for the diagnosis of CF because they may also be found in many types of chest disease.

How Is Cystic Fibrosis Treated?

ANTIBIOTIC THERAPY

Between 1979 and 1991, the age-related mortality rate for cystic fibrosis fell by 21 percent. Increases in survival rates in the last twenty-five years have been largely due to advances in antibiotic therapy.

Cystic fibrosis produces recurrent bouts of bacterial infection. Patients experience fever and increased cough and sputum production. When an exacerbation of CF occurs, the treatment of choice is antibiotic therapy given directly into a vein. This approach is needed to obtain adequate levels of the antibiotic in the clogged, damaged areas of the lungs. Oral antibiotic therapy is inadequate for treatment during these episodes.

Antibiotics have also been given by inhalation. This form of treatment appears most helpful when it is used as maintenance, preventive therapy after the acute episode has resolved. The FDA recently approved an inhalant form of the antibiotic tobramycin (Tobi), for the treatment of cystic fibrosis in patients at least six years old.

INHALATION THERAPY: DNASE (PULMOZYME)

A recent advance in the treatment of CF has been the development of a genetically engineered form of the human enzyme Dnase. This medication (Pulmozyme), which is delivered by inhalation, breaks up thick mucus, making it easier to clear by coughing. Patients receiving this enzyme have fewer infections and demonstrate improvement in pulmonary function.

BRONCHODILATORS AND STEROIDS

The use of bronchodilators and corticosteroids in CF patients is controversial. The results of bronchodilator therapy have been varied. Patients with overreactive bronchial tubes may respond to B-agonists or anti-cholinergic agents. In some patients, however, pulmonary function may be worse after the use of bronchodilators.

Patients with CF have been found to have an overactive immune response to infection. For this reason, corticosteroids have been given to small numbers of patients to reverse inflammation. The routine use of corticosteroids in the treatment of cystic fibrosis is not recommended.

PHYSICAL THERAPY

An essential part of the treatment of cystic fibrosis is the removal or drainage of mucus from the clogged and blocked air passages of the lungs. Physical therapy includes a technique known as postural drainage, as well as breathing exercises, percussion, and vibration; these must be performed several times a day by these patients. (These techniques are discussed in Chapter 7.)

Patients with CF have also been found to benefit from exercise training and conditioning. (An exercise test is usually done before the start of this form of therapy.)

OXYGEN THERAPY

In patients with advanced disease, oxygen therapy has reduced shortness of breath and prolonged life. Patients with milder forms of the disease may need oxygen therapy during exercise or sleep, when oxygen levels may fall.

NUTRITIONAL SUPPORT

In cystic fibrosis, the pancreas cannot function normally to provide the enzymes necessary to digest food, a condition known as pancreatic insufficiency. At the same time, patients with CF have increased nutritional needs due to infections and increased work of breathing.

Research has shown that nutritional supplementation improves lung function and extends survival in these patients.

The nutritional support of patients with CF includes the administration of pancreatic enzymes before each meal and snacks. A high-calorie, high-protein diet is recommended, as are vitamin supplements.

LUNG TRANSPLANTATION

Lung transplantation has been used in the treatment of cystic fibrosis. In patients with end-stage disease with heart and lung failure, both the heart and lungs have been transplanted. Double-lung transplant has also been used successfully in these patients. The five-year survival rate has reached more than 50 percent in some centers.

Transplantation results have improved steadily due to advances in antirejection drugs and surgical techniques. This approach continues to be limited by a lack of donors and long waiting lists.

THE FUTURE

Gene Therapy

The cloning of the cystic fibrosis gene has created optimism that a cure may be possible. Scientists have found that inactivated cold viruses may be used to carry normal genes to affected cells to correct the defect.

The early results of human trials of gene therapy in cystic fibrosis have been disappointing. Researchers, however, remain hopeful that this form of therapy may still provide a cure.

Drug Therapy

Another promising approach to the treatment of cystic fibrosis is the development of drugs that correct the defect in chloride transport across cell membranes. Several agents are being studied. One, CPX (8-cyclopentyl-a, 3-dipropylxanthine), is currently undergoing human trials.

CPX appears to bind to the defective CF protein and repair it to properly allow the transport of sodium and chloride to the outer cell surface.

Adults and Cystic Fibrosis

Although CF is a disease that primarily affects children, its many mutations have produced milder forms of the disorder, which may only be noted in adulthood. These patients are usually misdiagnosed as having chronic bronchitis, asthma, COPD, or bronchiectasis. Cystic fibrosis should be considered in any adult with recurrent episodes of chest infection.

An Achiever

Patients with cystic fibrosis are typically bright, articulate overachievers. I was privileged to care for Paul G. until his death at age forty-nine from cystic fibrosis. When I first met him, he already required continuous oxygen therapy and had signs of an enlarged heart. Despite this, Paul made it clear that he "was not going to let this disease run my life." He continued to work as a city official in New York through many hospitalizations and to speak and write extensively about surviving with cystic fibrosis. Unfortunately, his death came before the first heart-lung transplantation for cystic fibrosis had been performed. If this technique had been available during his lifetime, I am sure that he would have volunteered to be the first subject.

LUNG CANCER

Despite numerous public health warnings, lung cancer (bronchogenic carcinoma) remains a major health problem in the United States. In 1994, there were 172,000 newly diagnosed cases. In the same year, 153,000 Americans died of this disease. Lung cancer has been the leading cause of cancer deaths in men for the past four decades and has replaced breast cancer as the leading cause of cancer death in women in the past ten years. In addition to the striking human cost of this disease, the economic cost is enormous. Lung cancer–related costs are estimated to exceed ten billion dollars per year.

Causes of Lung Cancer

CIGARETTE SMOKING

A cause-and-effect relationship between lung cancer and cigarette smoking has been known to exist since the 1950s. It is estimated that more than 85 percent of lung cancer cases are due to cigarette smoking and are therefore preventable.

The active smoker's risk of developing lung cancer is directly related to a number of factors. The age the individual started smoking, the number of cigarettes smoked, the duration of smoking, and the tar and nicotine content of the cigarettes smoked appear to be the most important.

Compared with nonsmokers, smokers have a ten- to twenty-five-fold increased risk of developing lung cancer. When a smoker quits, however, there is a decline in cancer risk so that after ten to fifteen years, the risk of lung cancer approaches that of a lifelong nonsmoker. A recent report, however, suggests that smoking may permanently alter the smoker's DNA, creating a lifelong risk of developing lung cancer.

More than forty carcinogens have been found in cigarette smoke. The use of filter-tipped and low-tar and low-nicotine cigarettes may reduce exposure to some carcinogens, but smokers of these brands have increased the number of cigarettes smoked and inhale more deeply.

Secondhand Smoke

Nonsmokers are also at risk for lung cancer due to exposure to secondhand smoke. It has been estimated that 15 to 20 percent of lung cancer cases in nonsmokers are due to secondhand smoke. In 1993, the Environmental Protection Agency concluded that secondhand smoke is responsible for approximately three thousand lung cancer deaths per year in nonsmokers in the United States. (See Table 3.3 on page 69.)

OTHER CAUSES OF LUNG CANCER

Many other carcinogens that may cause lung cancer have been identified. Many of these materials were identified through the discovery of an increased number of lung cancer cases in workers involved in their production. These substances include nickel, arsenic, chromium, chloromethyl ether, vinyl chloride, and iron and steel used in founding.

Radon

The mining of radioactive ores was the first occupation to be linked to the development of lung cancer. Radon is a radiation-decay product that has been found sporadically in significant levels in residential dwellings in the United States. Recent studies conclude that it is an important cause of lung cancer in the general population. Radon may enter buildings through cracks or openings in the foundation and the highest levels are usually found in basements.

Asbestos

Asbestos is a well-known carcinogen that may cause lung cancer. Asbestos miners, shipbuilders, and textile workers exposed to asbestos have an increased risk of lung cancer compared with nonsmokers. This risk increases greatly if these individuals smoke cigarettes. The time period from the first exposure to asbestos and the development of lung cancer usually spans twenty to thirty years.

Asbestos may also cause another chest malignancy known as mesothelioma. This tumor arises on the pleura, the surface membrane that envelops the lung.

Types of Lung Cancer

Lung cancer is divided into four major types: adenocarcinoma, squamous cell carcinoma, small cell carcinoma, and large cell carcinoma. In terms of treatment options, lung cancer is commonly divided into small-cell and non–small cell carcinoma. All the major types of lung cancer are associated with cigarette smoking.

ADENOCARCINOMA

Adenocarcinoma is now the most common form of lung cancer, accounting for about one-third of all cases. Recent research suggests that the increase in the incidence of adenocarcinoma is directly related to the development of filter-tipped cigarettes with milder tobacco. With the development of these cigarettes, smokers have been forced to inhale more deeply to get the same amount of nicotine.

These tumors arise from the bronchial glands and are usually found in the outer portions of the lung. A subtype of adenocarcinoma is a form of lung cancer that grows within the air sacs, called alveolar cell carcinoma. This type of tumor may commonly mimic pneumonia.

SQUAMOUS CELL CARCINOMA

Squamous cell carcinoma accounts for 30 percent of all lung cancers. Prior to the increase in the incidence of adenocarcinoma, this cell type was the most common form of lung cancer. It has been directly linked to the use of unfiltered cigarettes, which produce harsher smoke and larger particles.

This tumor arises from damaged bronchial lining cells and typically grows closer to large bronchial tubes and the central chest structures. These structures include the large blood vessels, such as the aorta, the feeding passage (esophagus), and the heart. These structures are located within a central compartment of the chest, called the mediastinum. Many nerves and lymph glands are also located here.

SMALL CELL CARCINOMA

Small cell carcinoma represents 20 to 25 percent of lung cancer cases and is the most aggressive form of this disease, with the greatest propensity to spread (metastasize). This is a rapidly growing and spreading malignancy that arises in major bronchi. At the time of its discovery, small cell carcinoma usually has already spread to the lymph glands that surround the large bronchi and major blood vessels of the chest. It also has a tendency to produce hormonal substances that may produce total-body (non-respiratory) symptoms.

LARGE CELL CARCINOMA

Large cell carcinoma accounts for 15 to 20 percent of lung cancers. These tumors are usually found in the periphery of the lungs and resemble adenocarcinoma. Large cell cancers may spread directly to the outer chest wall or to the central lymph glands.

Symptoms of Lung Cancer

The symptoms of lung cancer vary according to the type of tumor. In small cell carcinoma, for example, the patient may actually first see a physician due to the spread of this malignancy outside the chest. Adenocarcinoma and large cell carcinoma grow more slowly but may also metastasize throughout the body. Squamous cell carcinoma tends to grow locally within the chest so that patients have symptoms resulting from a tumor invading the bronchial tube and surrounding region.

The growth of a lung cancer within a bronchial tube produces many symptoms. Patients often complain of cough and blood-streaked sputum. As the tumor grows and blocks the bronchial opening, the patient may note a wheeze and shortness of breath. Closure of a bronchus may lead to infection, making pneumonia another feature of lung cancer.

If the tumor is located near the outer portion of the lung, it may invade the pleural membrane and cause pain or fluid formation. Growth into the central chest structures may interfere with the nerve that controls the vocal cords and produce hoarseness or difficulty swallowing (dysphagia).

Lung cancers commonly spread outside the chest to the brain, liver, and bony skeleton by invading blood vessels and gaining access to the bloodstream. A common example is a patient who presents with what appears to be a stroke, only to be found to have a brain tumor that originated in the lung. Almost any organ of the body may be a site of distant spread of lung cancer. Within the chest, spread occurs either by direct invasion or through small channels called lymphatics, which connect groups of lymph glands.

Lung cancers often produce symptoms by producing hormonelike substances. These substances then act on the body to produce certain effects. For example, the development of a painful arthritis and the clubbing of the fingernails appears to be due, in part to a lung cancer producing a form of growth hormone. Small cell carcinoma frequently produces these hormonal substances.

Signs of Lung Cancer

The physical findings of lung cancer patients vary considerably and are not specific for this disease. The presence of clubbing of the fingers and swollen joints may signal the hormonal syndrome noted above. Clubbing may occur in other lung diseases when oxygen levels are reduced, and may also be present from birth.

Patients with an obstructed bronchus may have a wheeze that is localized to one lobe of the lung. Swollen, hard lymph nodes may be felt in the neck or under the arm in patients in which the disease has spread to glands outside of the chest. An enlarged, firm liver and signs of weight loss (cachexia) may suggest very advanced disease.

CHEST X-RAY AND CAT SCAN

The routine chest x-ray remains the best screening tool for detecting lung cancer, which typically appears as a rounded but irregular shadow (nodule) growing in the lung field. (See Fig. 3.6.) The human eye can

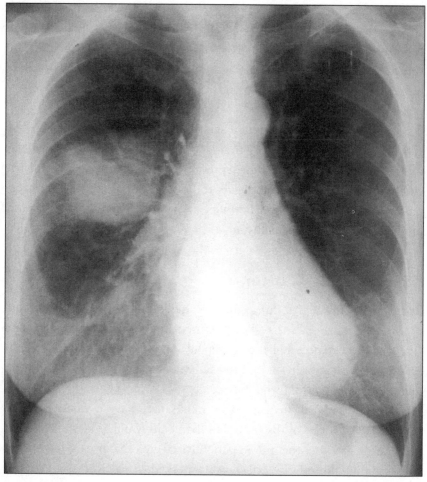

FIG. 3.6 CHEST X-RAY IN LUNG CANCER (appears as white shadow in upper right lung).

detect lesions that are 5 millimeters in diameter or greater in size. A nodule measuring 3 millimeters is rarely seen.

The lung cancer lesion has been described as having an irregular border. Although this contrasts with benign lesions, this feature does not differentiate a malignant lesion from a benign one.

If a lung cancer obstructs a bronchus, then the chest x-ray may reveal a collapsed lobe or lung. Fluid collection may appear on the x-ray of patients with spread to the pleural membrane. The chest x-ray may also show pneumonia in patients in whom an obstructed bronchus has allowed infection to set in. Alveolar cell carcinoma may mimic pneumonia on a chest x-ray because it grows within the lung's air sacs. Small cell carcinoma typically produces enlargement of the lymph nodes of the chest.

Although the routine chest x-ray can help diagnose lung cancer, the more detailed chest CAT scan is now used to better determine whether there has been spread within the chest. This process, called staging, is done routinely before treatment for lung cancer is initiated. CAT scanning may also be used for diagnosis when the results of a routine chest x-ray are equivocal. Despite further advances in technology, CAT scanning is not a perfect tool and the spread of lung cancer may not always be detected.

LABORATORY FINDINGS

There are no specific blood tests for lung cancer. A blood "marker" for lung cancer, however, may be available in the future. Carcinoembryonic antigen (CEA) is a blood marker that may be elevated in several cancers, including colon and lung. Unfortunately, it is also commonly increased in cigarette smokers who don't have lung cancer.

The abnormal blood results seen in lung cancer cases are usually due either to spread of the disease (liver or bone enzyme abnormalities) or hormonal syndromes produced by the results of the tumor (such as an elevated blood calcium level).

SPUTUM CYTOLOGY

The study of sputum for cancer cells is known as sputum cytology. This technique may provide an early diagnosis of this disease in selected patients. However, the results vary greatly and interpretation may be difficult with poor samples.

HIGH-RISK SCREENING

Lung cancer is difficult to cure unless it is detected at an early stage. For this reason, it is best to identify individuals who are at high risk and to monitor them closely for symptoms and signs of lung cancer. The high-risk group would be smokers aged forty-five and older. The best screening tool is a chest x-ray performed every six months. In selected patients, sputum cytology may also be helpful.

How Is Lung Cancer Diagnosed?

Once a chest lesion has been identified, it is necessary to obtain a specimen or biopsy. Sputum cytology may reveal lung cancer cells in patients who are expectorating phlegm.

A tissue diagnosis is usually obtained, either with the use of the fiberoptic bronchoscope or thin needle biopsy. In rare instances, surgery must be performed to obtain a diagnostic sample.

Treatment of Lung Cancer

The treatment of lung cancer is based on the cell type of the tumor, the stage of the disease, and the patient's health and lung function.

Once the diagnosis of lung cancer is made, the patient routinely must undergo CAT scanning of the brain, abdomen, and pelvis, a bone scan, and pulmonary function tests. Another technique of producing an image, Magnetic Resonance Imaging (MRI), may also detect the spread.

The Stages of Lung Cancer

Lung cancer is classified by stages to allow the physician to determine the best treatment option. In general, Stages I and II are smaller tumors that have not spread locally or distantly. These tumors are treated by surgically removing them. Stage III tumors are larger and have spread locally, not distantly. Some of these tumors can be removed surgically, but many are inoperable and must be treated with radiation or chemotherapy. Stage IV tumors have spread from the lung to distant sites and are inoperable. These advanced tumors are treated with chemotherapy.

At the time of discovery, more than 70 percent of lung cancers are either Stage III or IV. The definition of a cancer cure is a patient who survives five years from the time of diagnosis. Patients with small tumors that have not spread (Stage I) have a 60 to 70 percent five-year survival rate whereas only 2 percent of patients with spread to other organs (Stage IV) survive five years.

SURGERY FOR LUNG CANCER

Surgery is the most effective treatment for lung cancer. It is the only option that may consistently provide a cure for this disease.

Patients undergoing surgery must have adequate lung function to permit removal (resection) of the diseased portion, as well as a healthy margin of the surrounding tissue. The most common procedure is to remove the tumor and surrounding tissue (lobectomy). Removal of a smaller portion of lung (wedge resection) may be performed in selected patients who have reduction of lung function as determined by pulmonary function testing. Complete removal of a lung (pneumonectomy) may be necessary in more advanced cases. At the time of surgery, the surgeon routinely examines and removes lymph nodes from the chest to determine the spread.

Surgery for lung cancer requires general anesthesia. In the population greater than seventy-five years of age, the risk of complications from general anesthesia, including stroke and heart attack, increases. For this reason, elderly patients with lung cancer and significant heart or circulatory disease may be judged to be at high risk for surgery. In these patients, other treatment options may be suggested.

RADIATION THERAPY

Radiation therapy is an effective means of shrinking smaller tumors but does not provide a cure for lung cancer except in extremely rare cases. It may be useful in shrinking a tumor that is blocking a bronchial tube or causing severe bone pain. In selected patients, radiation may also be combined with surgery or chemotherapy.

Radiation is given over a period of weeks with a schedule of treatments for five days per week. This gradual process of administering radiation in small doses is performed so as to minimize side effects. These treatments are painless and take minutes. Side effects may include nausea and loss of appetite. These effects usually clear up about one month after radiation therapy has completed. Long-term effects are uncommon but include cough and shortness of breath due to lung damage.

CHEMOTHERAPY FOR LUNG CANCER

Chemotherapy is the injection into the body of potent chemicals that are capable of destroying lung cancer cells. However, these powerful drugs cannot cure lung cancer. Chemotherapy, however, may extend survival.

Chemotherapy is most effective in small cell lung cancer and may prolong life for one to three years. The results in non–small cell cases are mixed, with less than 50 percent of patients achieving a significant response.

Chemotherapy is given over a period of months in cycles that are separated by three to four weeks. Side effects include nausea, reduced immunity to infection, low blood counts (anemia), fatigue, and hair and weight loss. In all patients receiving chemotherapy, the prolonged survival must be weighed against the quality of life achieved.

Choosing No Treatment

The decision to treat lung cancer is made after diagnosis and staging are determined. When faced with the options of surgery, radiation, and chemotherapy, many patients may decline treatment. These individuals have Stage III or IV disease and wish to avoid the adverse effects of chemotherapy.

In the elderly patient with lung cancer, decision making must weigh the risks of treatment, as well as life expectancy. Many patients choose not to be treated. Selected patients, however, may undergo surgical resection if preliminary testing shows that they are not at high risk for complications. In this group of patients, underlying heart, lung, and kidney disease may contradict any form of treatment.

THE NATURAL COURSE

Patients who do not undergo any form of treatment or who fail to respond when treatment is given experience the effects of growth of their malignancy. The nature of these effects is determined by the growth rate, stage, and type of lung cancer. In patients with non–small-cell carcinoma, the growth rate may be slow so that these individuals may survive for extended periods.

Supportive treatment, which includes pain medication, nutritional support, and possibly oxygen therapy, is directed by the physician.

Additional support may be provided by a number of agencies. (See the appendix.)

A Story of Survival

Kevin L. is now fifty-two years old. I met Kevin sixteen years earlier for complaints of shortness of breath. He was a heavy cigarette smoker and I found that he already had emphysema with large cysts in both lungs. I recommended bronchodilator therapy and he resolved to quit smoking. At age thirty-eight, Kevin returned with complaints of cough and fever, and his chest x-ray revealed a lung mass. A needle biopsy revealed a non–small cell carcinoma. Preliminary work-up revealed Stage III disease; one surgeon declined to operate. A cancer specialist suggested that Kevin start chemotherapy, and gave him six months to live.

I decided to push for surgery and Kevin agreed. He resolved to survive and to come back to tell the surgeon and cancer specialist how wrong they were. Dr. Naels Martini at Memorial Sloan-Kettering Hospital agreed that surgery was possible. Kevin underwent an operation on his "good" lung to remove cysts and improve his lung function. Four weeks later a lobectomy was performed to remove the tumor mass. One month later Kevin developed a change in his vision and a CAT scan discovered three metastatic brain tumors. He underwent radiation therapy to the brain, followed by surgery that could find no residual tumor.

Less than a month after brain surgery, a chest CAT scan showed that his chest tumor had recurred. Due to his emphysema and previous surgery, a pneumonectomy was not possible, and Kevin underwent a procedure to implant radioactive seeds next to his tumor. This technique delivered a large amount of radiation that could not have been safely given by the usual method. Throughout the entire, difficult time period, which included three operations, and brain and chest radiation therapy, Kevin remained determined to survive.

Fourteen years after the diagnosis of inoperable lung cancer, Kevin is working and counsels cancer patients in his spare time. Although his story is the exception, it says that survival is possible.

FOLLOWING THE AIRWAYS

The bronchial tubes branch many times before reaching the lung's air sacs. The smallest bronchial tube is called the terminal bronchiole; it opens into the alveolar sacs. In this chapter, several important diseases that affect primarily the bronchial tubes have been discussed. Many of these diseases, such as emphysema, also affect the air sacs of the lung. In the next chapter, diseases that affect primarily the alveoli are discussed.

4

DISEASES OF THE AIR SACS

INTERSTITIAL LUNG DISEASES

The lung's air sacs are lined by columns of cells that assist in maintaining the normal lung structure. These cells are also capable of repairing lung damage but are vulnerable to injury. The walls between the air sacs contain many other types of cells, as well as a supporting tissue, called collagen, and the capillary blood vessels. This tissue between the air sacs is called the interstitium, and diseases that affect this vital area are often called interstitial lung diseases. Although this term suggests that the disease process is confined to the space between the alveoli, these disorders usually involve the air sacs as well.

As many as 130 breathing disorders are known to affect the lung's air sacs and interstitium. Many do not have known causes and are called idiopathic. Although these disorders are diverse and their courses vary, they share many common properties. They typically produce shortness of breath, which is first noted after exertion. Some patients may also have a dry, persistent cough. Chest x-rays commonly show diffuse lung changes, while pulmonary function tests reveal loss of lung capacity.

Many patients with this form of lung disease may ignore their symptoms. Some patients only seek medical attention when symptoms become severe. This denial of illness is detrimental, since treatment of these lung diseases is only effective if given early in the course of the illness. As interstitial lung disease (ILD) progresses, the lung tissue thickens and becomes stiff, increasing the work of breathing. Many patients with ILD experience severe air hunger and require oxygen therapy.

All of these disorders begin with inflammation. When it involves the air sacs it is called alveolitis. This form of lung injury may lead to permanent lung damage or scarring of lung tissue (fibrosis). In this chapter, two of the most common interstitial lung diseases, pulmonary fibrosis and sarcoidosis, will be discussed.

Pulmonary Fibrosis

In pulmonary fibrosis, the air sacs of the lung are permanently destroyed and replaced by scar tissue. The tissue between the sacs (interstitium), as well as the small capillary blood vessels are also destroyed. In patients with severe disease, the architecture of the lung is severely distorted, making normal alveoli difficult to find under the microscope. The only beneficial treatments for patients with advanced disease may be oxygen and lung transplantation.

WHAT CAUSES PULMONARY FIBROSIS?

In the majority of patients with pulmonary fibrosis, the physician can identify the source. This is particularly true of patients who acquire this illness through exposure to materials at home or in the workplace. In many individuals, however, the cause of fibrosis is unknown.

All cases of fibrosis appear to begin with an injury to the cells that line the air sacs. Once alveoli are injured (alveolitis), a repair process is initiated. If the injury is unchecked, then the alveolitis and attempts at repair result in destruction and scarring of the alveoli. If the injury can be interrupted or the inflammation suppressed, then fibrosis can be prevented.

What Precipitates the Injury?

Many mechanisms produce the initial lung injury. In some cases, a foreign substance, such as coal dust, is inhaled into the lung and creates the initial injury. Infections, such as tuberculosis, activate immune cells that lead to inflammation and injury. The immune system may also cause lung injury by producing antibodies that attack the lining cells of the alveoli. In all these instances, the lung injury may be augmented by the stimulation of repair cells, which are then drawn into the damaged area.

SPECIFIC CAUSES OF PULMONARY FIBROSIS

Many causes of pulmonary fibrosis have been identified. Table 4.1 lists some of the most common sources. A discussion of each category is beyond the scope of this book, but a few important sources of fibrosis will be discussed.

Drugs

The ability of certain medications to produce fibrosis of the lungs has been recognized for years. In most instances, this adverse effect is produced gradually over a period of months and is related to the amount of medication ingested.

Amiodarone (Cordarone)

Amiodarone (Cordarone) is a widely used cardiac medication that controls abnormal heart rhythms. Since a case report in 1980, physicians have known that amiodarone may produce pulmonary fibrosis. The frequency of this adverse effect has varied between 4 and 27 percent in major research studies. Patients typically develop cough and exhibit shortness of breath over a period of months. The most striking risk factor for the development of pulmonary fibrosis from amiodarone is the day-to-day dosage administered. Patients receiving more than 400 milligrams per day are clearly at an increased risk of developing this side effect.

Methotrexate

Methotrexate is widely prescribed in the treatment of rheumatoid arthritis. This medication is also used in the treatment of many forms of cancer, as well as for other diseases that involve the immune system. It has also been used extensively in the treatment of severe psoriasis.

Approximately 7 percent of patients receiving methotrexate will develop lung toxicity. This reaction may take the form of a pneumonia but is more commonly manifested as pulmonary fibrosis.

TABLE 4.1 COMMON CAUSES OF PULMONARY FIBROSIS

---

1. Known Causes
    A. Environmental and occupational: dusts, gases, and fumes
    B. Drugs
        a. Amiodarone (Cordarone)
        b. Methotrexate
        c. Anticancer agents
    C. Infectious agents
        a. Tuberculosis
        b. Fungi
    D. Allergic or Hypersensitivity pneumonitis

2. Unknown Causes
    A. Idiopathic pulmonary fibrosis
    B. Sarcoidosis

Anticancer Agents

In addition to methotrexate, several anticancer agents have been shown to cause pulmonary fibrosis. Some of the most common are bleomycin, carmustine (BCNU), mitomycin, and busulfan. This list increases almost daily as newer agents are introduced for the treatment of malignancy.

When a cancer patient who is receiving one of these medications has shortness of breath, the difficulty may be attributed to the underlying malignancy and not the drug. To distinguish malignancy from drug reaction, a careful analysis of x-rays, breathing tests, and even lung biopsy may be necessary.

Occupational and Environmental Sources of Fibrosis

The workplace and the home may allow exposure to substances that when inhaled produce pulmonary fibrosis. The lung disease produced is often linked to the patient's occupation, such as "bird breeder's lung," whereby inhalation of bird proteins from dropping or feathers produces lung inflammation and ultimately fibrosis. The disease may also occur in the home, as in "hot-tub lung," where inhalation of mold spores produces lung damage. Some of the most common sources of fibrosis are discussed below and are listed in Table 4.2 on p. 142.

Asbestos

Asbestos is an almost indestructible fiber whose usefulness was recognized as long as 4,500 years ago in pottery making. Today, asbestos exists in thousands of materials, including cement products, floor tiles, roofing, and insulation. Lung disease (asbestosis) as a result of the inhalation of asbestos particles has been recognized for years.

The development and severity of pulmonary fibrosis as a result of asbestos depends on the amount inhaled, as well as duration of exposure. Small exposures over many years may have the same impact as a brief, intense exposure.

Strict government standards to prevent asbestos-induced lung disease have been implemented. Asbestos products now "lock in" the fibers to prevent them from being inhaled. Danger from asbestos, however, currently exists from exposure to old, crumbling asbestos-containing materials. Caution must be taken in removing or destroying these materials.

Other durable fibers, including talc, glass, and ceramic, may also cause pulmonary fibrosis.

Silica

Silica is the predominant component of the Earth's crust, so it may be encountered in any form of mining, quarrying, or tunneling operation. Sandblasters, pottery workers, and foundry workers are also frequently exposed to silica.

When small particles of silica are inhaled into the alveoli, inflammation and subsequently, fibrosis result. The severity of scarring depends on the amount inhaled and the length of time that the individual is exposed. The damage produced may vary, from massive destruction of the lung to mild scarring.

Silicosis is a preventable disease that requires specific control measures. Dust control, masks, ventilation, and the wetting down of mines have been useful in the prevention of this disease.

Gases

Noxious gases and mists may injure the delicate tissue lining the bronchial tubes and alveoli. The most commonly encountered irritant gases are chlorine, phosgene, ammonia, sulfur dioxide, and nitrogen dioxide.

Nitrogen Dioxide

Nitrogen dioxide (NO_2), a reddish-brown gas with a pungent odor, may produce severe lung irritation and damage. The degree of injury is dependent on the concentration of the gas and the duration of exposure. Most injuries from NO_2 occur as the result of industrial exposures. Nitrogen dioxide is produced in the manufacture of explosives, dyes, lacquers, and during arc welding. This gas is also a common air pollutant, which may exacerbate COPD and asthma.

Nitrogen dioxide may also be produced by the oxidation of nitrates in green plants. Farm workers who entered silos where these plants were stored have suffered NO_2 inhalation. This illness is often called "silo-filler's disease."

▓ Organic Dusts

Pulmonary fibrosis may occur in susceptible individuals after exposure to a large variety and increasing number of organic materials. These materials are primarily bacteria, fungi, and animal proteins. When a susceptible individual inhales these substances, a reaction occurs in the lung as many types of immune cells are activated. The initial lung reaction may mimic pneumonia, with the presence of fever and cough, but repeated exposures may gradually produce fibrosis and the primary symptom of shortness of breath.

This disorder is often called "hypersensitivity pneumonitis," but is usually linked to the patient's occupation ("farmer's lung") or the place of exposure ("sauna-taker's disease"). Table 4.2 lists some examples, as well as suspected irritating agents. Not everyone who is exposed to the offending substance develops this disease.

The diagnosis of hypersensitivity pneumonitis is made from the combination of known exposure to an offending substance and x-ray findings, laboratory studies, and lung biopsy. In most patients with this disease, an antibody to the irritating substance (antigen) is found in the blood. In some instances, the diagnosis is made through a challenge test in which the patient is intentionally exposed to the antigen and observed for the development of a lung reaction.

Treatment of this disorder includes avoidance of the offending substance. This may be as simple as disposing of a contaminated humidifier or finding another home for a bird. In many patients, avoidance may be the only treatment necessary. In patients with severe symptoms and lung reaction, corticosteroids are usually administered.

Farmer's Lung

Farmer's lung develops from repeated exposure to moldy hay. In most cases, fever is noted in the evening after a day's work. Most patients only seek medical attention after several months or years of shortness of breath.

It is estimated that up to 8 percent of farmers may develop this disorder. In 60 to 80 percent of patients, antibodies to molds *(Thermoactinomyces vulgaris, Faenia rectivirgula)* are found in blood testing.

TABLE 4.2 EXAMPLES OF HYPERSENSITIVITY PNEUMONITIS

Disease Name	Source of Antigen
Farmer's lung	Moldy hay
Malt-worker's lung	Contaminated barley
Humidifier lung	Contamination of humidifier
Coffee-worker's lung	Green coffee beans
Sauna-taker's disease	Sauna water
Hot-tub lung	Mold on ceiling
Saxophone lung	Saxophone mouthpiece
Pigeon-breeder's disease	Pigeon droppings
Bird-fancier's lung	Bird products
Dove-pillow's lung	Bird feathers
Wine-grower's lung	Mold on grapes

Corticosteroids are usually required for the treatment of farmer's lung. Possible methods to prevent relapse of this disease include improving hay-making techniques, converting bedding from straw to wood chips, improving barn ventilation, and wearing protective masks. With these preventive steps, the patient can usually remain on the farm.

Humidifier Lung

Humidifiers are increasingly found in the home and workplace. Humidifier lung results from the moldy contamination of the water reservoir. This problem may occur in both warm and cool air humidifiers, with inhalation of a variety of mold spores contained in water droplets.

Patients typically present to the physician with fever, cough, and shortness of breath and are often initially treated for pneumonia. On careful questioning, the patient will note the use of a humidifier. Antibodies against the molds are usually found in the blood.

Humidifier lung can be prevented by frequent cleaning of the humidifier. The reservoir water should be changed daily. In most cases of humidifier lung, treatment consists of avoidance of further mold exposure. A brief course of corticosteroids may also be necessary.

A Case of Bird-Fancier's Lung

JT was a sixty-eight-year-old former postal worker who I encountered during my pulmonary fellowship at Bellevue Hospital. He had been admitted with cough, fever, and shortness of breath, and his chest x-ray strongly suggested interstitial lung disease. Blood-gas analysis revealed a lowered oxygen level. During his initial interview, I asked if he had any pets, especially birds; he said no.

The patient underwent lung biopsy, which revealed the changes of hypersensitivity pneumonitis. Before I had a chance to explain the findings to him, I received a call from his wife inquiring as to the results. I told her that although we now knew the type of lung disease affecting her husband, the cause was still unknown. I was surprised when she said, "What about those damn birds?" It seems that JT had hidden the fact that he kept songbirds, fearing that he would have to give them up if they were found to be the source of his illness. (He later mentioned that his wife did not share his love of birds.) The patient was treated with corticosteroids and advised to find a new home for the songbirds. His wife assured me that he would.

IDIOPATHIC PULMONARY FIBROSIS

In approximately 50 percent of patients with pulmonary fibrosis, the cause is unknown. Despite the lack of a known cause, idiopathic pulmonary fibrosis (IPF) is a distinct illness with characteristic physical and laboratory findings. IPF is now thought to be more common, occurring in nearly sixty individuals per one hundred thousand of the population in the United States.

IPF strikes both sexes equally, usually in the fifth to sixth decade of life. Current research indicates that IPF begins with an inciting injury to the lung's air sacs. This injury draws inflammatory and immune cells to the alveoli, causing alveolitis. Despite the fact that the inciting agent, which may be viral, appears to leave the lung, the alveolitis continues and ultimately destroys the air sacs.

Once established, IPF progresses relentlessly in most patients and proves fatal in 50 percent of them within five years. Treatment of IPF is only effective if it is initiated in the earliest stages. Unfortunately, many patients delay medical attention until they have passed through the earliest phases of IPF.

Symptoms of Idiopathic Pulmonary Fibrosis

Progressive shortness of breath is the most common symptom of IPF patients. In the early stages, breathlessness is only noted with exertion, but as the disease progresses, patients find themselves out of breath with almost any activity. Many patients interpret the first signs of air hunger as "being out of shape" and delay medical attention until they are much worse.

A dry, persistent cough is also a frequent symptom of IPF. In some individuals, cough may be the dominant symptom. This cough rarely produces much sputum and may be nearly continuous, and grow worse with speech. In taking the history of patients with IPF, it is common to find that cough frequently interrupts speech.

IPF patients may occasionally note excessive fatigue, fever, night sweats, and weight loss. Pain in muscles and joints may also occur and prompt consultation.

Taking the Medical History in IPF

It is important to record a detailed medical history in patients suspected of having IPF. A thorough review of the patient's occupation and environment should be performed. Patients may not consider a pet, humidifier, or hot tub a potential source of lung disease and unless questioned, may fail to mention their presence in the home. As the list of causes of hypersensitivity pneumonitis grows, it is important to consider any occupation or activity as a potential source of disease.

A detailed drug history is also vital and must include illegal drugs, including marijuana and cocaine. An unfortunate practice of the drug culture is the snorting of drugs. This quick nasal inhalation allows drugs and the fillers they are mixed with to enter the lungs and produce interstitial lung disease.

Signs of Idiopathic Pulmonary Fibrosis

The physical findings of patients with IPF vary depending on the stage of the disease. A more rapid rate of breathing is common, and those with advanced stages of this disease take small, short breaths. A striking finding is the presence of snapping sounds, called crackles. In IPF, these sounds occur in virtual showers and resemble the sound produced by separating Velcro.

Clubbing of the nails occurs in 30 to 75 percent of patients with IPF but is not specific to this disorder. In advanced disease, the physical examination may also reveal cyanosis, as well as signs of heart failure, often indicated by swelling of the legs.

How Is IPF Diagnosed?

The diagnosis of IPF is made by identifying characteristic physical, laboratory, x-ray, and lung-biopsy findings. At the same time, the physician must exclude known causes, as well as other diseases of unknown cause that also produce fibrosis of the lung.

Chest X-Ray Findings in IPF

After the patient's history is taken and the physical examination completed, the physician turns to the chest x-ray, and increasingly to the chest CAT scan in patients suspected of having IPF.

Up to 10 percent of patients with interstitial disease, however, have a normal chest x-ray. In the majority, the x-ray is abnormal and the findings may be striking. In early stages of IPF, the normally clear lung fields become hazy. This finding has been associated with the alveolitis phase of this disease. As the lung is further damaged, lacy line shadows are seen, which represent thickened and damaged walls of the alveoli. (See Fig. 4.1.) The final stage of pulmonary fibrosis produces a striking picture, called honeycombing, in which the x-ray reveals small cystlike shadows throughout the lung fields.

Chest CAT scanning best demonstrates the x-ray findings of IPF and has become an excellent diagnostic tool. No form of x-ray, however, can substitute for a tissue biopsy.

Laboratory Findings of IPF

There is no specific blood test for IPF. It is important, however, to use laboratory testing to help exclude other causes of pulmonary fibrosis, such as hypersensitivity pneumonitis.

Laboratory analysis of the cells within the lung is useful in the diagnosis of interstitial lung diseases. These cells are obtained through the use of the fiberoptic bronchoscope. In this procedure, which is called bronchoalveolar lavage, the physician rinses the lung to obtain cellular material.

Pulmonary Function Testing in IPF

Pulmonary function tests are often revealing in patients with IPF. In the early stages of this disease, spirometry and lung volumes may be normal. The diffusion capacity is often reduced, however, due to injury to the air sacs and the damage to capillary blood vessels. As the disease progresses, lung volumes fall.

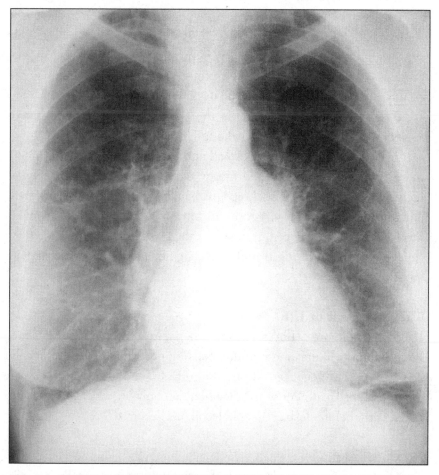

FIG. 4.1 CHEST X-RAY IN IDIOPATHIC PULMONARY FIBROSIS (appears as lacy pattern in lower lungs).

Advanced IPF often produces profound drops in oxygen levels, so that patients often require oxygen therapy. In the early stages, oxygen levels may be normal at rest but decrease with exertion. Patients with IPF have stiff lungs and breathe rapidly, making carbon dioxide levels low. An elevated carbon dioxide level in a patient with IPF is an ominous finding that signals an end stage of this progressive disease.

Lung Biopsy: The Final Step

Biopsy of the lung is the most revealing diagnostic step in the evaluation of patients suspected of having IPF. In general, every patient with IPF should have a tissue biopsy. In advanced disease, where biopsy may present significant risk to the life of the patient, the physician may rely on the information gained from the tests previously noted.

Biopsies may be obtained via the fiberoptic bronchoscope or by surgery ("open"). Unfortunately, the lung tissue samples obtained by the less invasive bronchoscopy are small and may be inadequate for a definite diagnosis. The open lung biopsy obtained through a small chest incision is the procedure of choice. By using a video camera to guide the cutting instrument, a surgeon can obtain a larger sample from an involved area. This procedure must be done while the patient is asleep (under general anesthesia) and poses significant risk in patients with advanced disease.

The Treatment of IPF

Idiopathic pulmonary fibrosis begins when a lung injury produces alveolar inflammation, drawing immune cells into the air sacs of the lung. If this process is unchecked, destruction of alveoli and interstitial tissue develops. The treatment of this disorder can only be effective if it is initiated early, before destruction of alveoli has occurred.

Corticosteroids

Corticosteroids are the most effective treatment for IPF. Steroids work by reducing inflammation in the air sacs. To be effective, this therapy must be initiated early in the course of the disease. Treatment is generally given for one year, beginning at a high dose, with slow tapering after the first three months. Unfortunately, corticosteroids may not be beneficial, especially if given too late.

Other drugs that affect the immune system have been used alone or in combination with corticosteroids. These include cyclophosphamide, methotrexate, and azathioprine. None of these agents has been found to be superior to corticosteroids.

Oxygen Therapy

Patients with IPF often have low blood oxygen levels. These patients benefit from oxygen therapy. In some patients, oxygen levels are adequate at rest but drop precipitously with exertion. Portable oxygen units allow the patient to increase activity and thus improve their quality of life.

Lung Transplantation

The natural course of IPF is typically a relentless progression, ultimately ending with severe lung damage. Patients who have had no response to drug therapy should be considered for lung transplantation. Significant progress in lung transplantation has been made, making this extreme option an accepted form of treatment for IPF and other end-stage lung diseases.

Single lung transplantation has been performed since 1983, and has become the procedure of choice for patients with end-stage IPF and emphysema.

Transplantation is limited by two major factors: the scarcity of donors and the possibility of rejection of the transplanted organ. Improvements in antirejection medications are continuing. Unfortunately, many patients die while awaiting a suitable donor.

SARCOIDOSIS

Sarcoidosis is total-body disease of diverse manifestations that may cause pulmonary fibrosis. The hallmark of this breathing disorder is the production in body tissues of an inflammatory lesion called noncaseating granuloma. Sarcoidosis appears to develop when a susceptible individual is exposed to a substance capable of provoking an exaggerated immune system reaction. The immune reaction is driven by stimulated cells that produce a characteristic form of inflammation, called granuloma. Almost any organ in the body may be a target of the stimulated immune cells so that sarcoidosis has a variety of physical manifestations. In a small percentage of patients, inflammation in these organs may progress to fibrosis and permanent damage.

Who Gets Sarcoidosis?

Sarcoidosis occurs worldwide, affecting people of all races, ages, and both sexes. This disease has a predilection to occur in people younger than age forty, in large cities, and in certain ethnic and racial groups. In the United States, sarcoidosis occurs in eleven Caucasians per a hundred thousand, and in thirty-six African-Americans per a hundred thousand.

Race also appears to affect how sarcoidosis manifests itself. In Caucasians, few symptoms occur; the disease may be discovered on a routine x-ray. In African-Americans, the disease often produces more acute problems, such as fever and inflammation of the eye (uveitis).

What Causes Sarcoidosis?

The cause of sarcoidosis remains unknown but numerous theories abound. This is not unexpected in view of the many organs that may be attacked by the disease, as well as the diversity of manifestations.

The discovery of a cause of sarcoidosis has been complicated by the fact that noncaseating granuloma, the microscopic lesion associated with the disease, may be found in other disease entities as well. Granuloma represents an inflammatory reaction, so it has been seen in a variety of infections, including tuberculosis. For many years, sarcoidosis was, in fact, thought to be a form of tuberculosis.

Many features of cases of sarcoidosis suggest that it is caused by an environmental agent. Clusters of cases have occurred among groups that live together, such as nurses and firefighters. Experts speculate that sarcoidosis is caused by a germ or pollutant that can be inhaled.

A Genetic Link

Genetic factors also appear to play a role in the development of sar-coidosis. Research suggests that sarcoidosis develops in individuals who are genetically predisposed to overreact to substances that are inhaled, producing an immune response that causes granuloma.

Symptoms of Sarcoidosis

The symptoms of sarcoidosis are variable. Most patients develop non-specific symptoms, such as fatigue, fever, loss of appetite, and weight loss. Many patients report shortness of breath, cough, and chest dis-comfort. Inflammation of the eye (conjunctivitis) may also be seen.

In 20 to 50 percent of patients with sarcoidosis, an acute illness develops. These patients have an unusual skin lesion, called erythema nodosum, in which tender, red bumps appear on the shin area of both legs. These patients also have pain in their joints (arthralgia) and swollen lymph glands on their chest x-rays.

Many patients with sarcoidosis do not have symptoms. In these individuals, the disease is first noted on a routine chest x-ray.

Physical Findings in Sarcoidosis

Sarcoidosis may affect a number of different organ systems of the body. Almost every sarcoidosis patient has involvement of the respiratory sys-tem. The most common manifestation is inflammation of the air sacs, producing signs of interstitial lung disease (crackles) on examination. Sarcoidosis may also involve the bronchial tubes and mimic asthma by producing narrowing of the air passages and causing wheezing. Patients have been called asthmatic, only to be subsequently found to have sar-coidosis. Sarcoidosis may also involve the upper respiratory tract, pro-ducing nasal and sinus obstruction due to inflammation. Approximately 25 percent of patients will have skin lesions, which include the tender nodules of erythema nodosum. Other lesions may occur in scars and tat-toos. Swollen lymph glands are common in sarcoidosis but are not spe-cific to this disease. Inflammation of the eye may also take many forms, often producing blurred vision, tearing, and sensitivity to light (photo-phobia).

Making the Diagnosis of Sarcoidosis

A definitive test for sarcoidosis has yet to be developed. Instead, the physician assembles characteristic findings of the disease, while excluding other illnesses that may also produce granuloma formation.

▓ The Chest X-Ray

Sarcoidosis is often first suspected by the review of a routine chest x-ray. One of the most common patterns of disease is the enlargement of the lymph glands that surround the windpipe and bronchial tubes. (See Fig. 4.2.) In sarcoidosis, physicians see a striking, symmetrical enlargement of these glands so that the right- and left-sided lymph nodes are mirror images of each other. Although this pattern is highly suggestive of sarcoidosis, it is not specific to this disease and may be seen in lymphoma, a malignancy of the lymph system.

Sarcoidosis may also cause interstitial disease so that the chest x-ray may be similar to that of idiopathic pulmonary fibrosis. (See Fig. 4.3.) In end-stage disease, honeycombing may be seen. The combination of enlarged lymph glands with interstitial disease certainly suggests sarcoidosis. Chest CAT scanning may be used to better visualize the interstitial component of sarcoidosis and to confirm enlargement of lymph glands.

▓ Laboratory Studies

There is no specific laboratory test for sarcoidosis, but certain findings may suggest this disease. The blood of patients with sarcoidosis often reveals elevation of protein, calcium, and liver enzymes.

One laboratory test, called angiotensin converting enzyme level (ACE), may be elevated in up to 75 percent of patients with sarcoidosis. Unfortunately, this test has been found to be elevated in other illnesses and cannot be used to confirm the diagnosis. Once the ACE level is found to be elevated, however, it may be used as a barometer of the disease. In a patient with proven sarcoidosis, who is treated with corticosteroids, for example, the elevated ACE will often decrease, reflecting a decrease in the activity of the illness.

A skin test known as the Kviem-Siltzbach test for the diagnosis of sarcoidosis has been used by a handful of medical centers. This test is performed by injecting under the skin material from the spleen or lymph nodes of a patient with known sarcoidosis. After six weeks, the injected area is biopsied, looking for granuloma formation. This test is not available in most medical centers and is not approved by the FDA for general use.

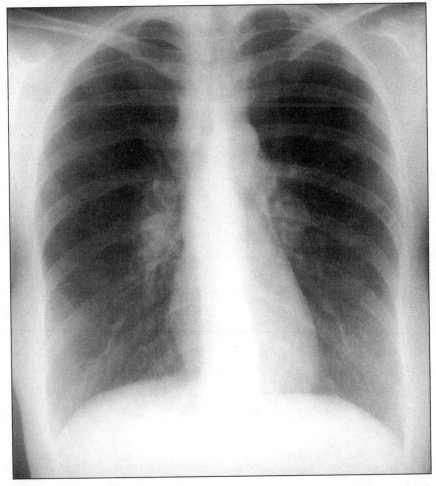

FIG. 4.2 CHEST X-RAY IN SARCOIDOSIS (enlarged lymph glands surround windpipe).

■ Pulmonary Function Tests

Abnormalities in pulmonary function testing are not specific for the diagnosis of sarcoidosis. This testing is important, however, in evaluating these patients and may be the deciding factor in determining treatment.

Patients with inflammation of the bronchial tubes due to sarcoidosis will often demonstrate airflow obstruction on spirometry. The use of

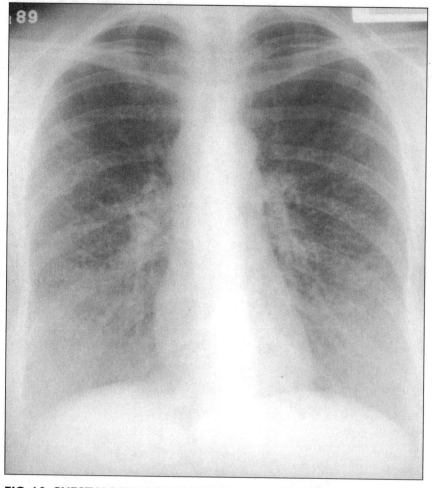

FIG. 4.3 CHEST X-RAY IN SARCOIDOSIS WITH FIBROSIS
(note resemblance to Fig. 4.1).

bronchodilator medication in these patients may result in improvement, suggesting a diagnosis of asthma. Lung volume measurement may be normal or reduced in those patients with interstitial involvement. A reduction in the diffusion capacity may also reflect interstitial inflammation due to sarcoidosis.

Exercise testing may be revealing in patients with sarcoidosis with interstitial involvement. These patients may have normal oxygen levels at rest, which decrease on exercise testing. This decrease often correlates with the shortness of breath these patients experience with exertion.

Biopsy: The Ultimate Test

In the final diagnosis of sarcoidosis, a tissue sample that reveals the characteristic noncaseating granuloma must be obtained. At the same time, the tissue sample must not contain evidence of any known source of granuloma formation, such as tuberculosis or fungal organisms. The physician can only be confident of the diagnosis after excluding all known causes of this type of inflammation.

What Type of Biopsy Is Best?

Because sarcoidosis may involve a number of organs, tissue samples may be obtained from a variety of sources. One of the most accessible and least invasive is a biopsy of a skin lesion. Fiberoptic bronchoscopy with biopsy is also a commonly used method to obtain tissue samples for the diagnosis of sarcoidosis. The physician may obtain with a fiberoptic instrument samples of the lining of the bronchial tubes, as well as the interstitium and air sacs. This procedure is performed with a local anesthetic and sedation, and is commonly done in the outpatient setting.

In selected patients, the diagnosis of sarcoidosis may be made through biopsy of other involved areas of the body, such as lymph glands, the conjunctiva of the eye, and the liver.

How Is Sarcoidosis Treated?

The drug of choice for the treatment of sarcoidosis is a corticosteroid. As in the patients with IPF, if treatment is to be successful, it must be given before the development of pulmonary fibrosis. Cortico-steroids are typically taken orally over a period of months, with a gradual reduction in dosage.

In certain types of sarcoidosis, steroids may also be given in other forms. Patients with milder forms of eye involvement may be treated with a steroid eyedrop, for example. In patients with bronchial inflammation from sarcoidosis, a topical steroid spray may be successful in controlling cough and shortness of breath. Sarcoid skin lesions may also be treated with local injection of corticosteroid.

Although the treatment of sarcoidosis with corticosteroids is usually effective, up to 25 percent of patients with more advanced sarcoidosis will relapse after corticosteroids are withdrawn. These patients may require long-term treatment and must be closely monitored for adverse effects of corticosteroids.

Who Should Be Treated?

In view of the favorable course of many patients with sarcoidosis, the decision to administer treatment must be well founded. In 60 to 80 percent of sarcoidosis patients with early stages that involve only the lymph glands of the chest, spontaneous resolution of the disease occurs. In patients with interstitial disease, this percentage drops to 30 to 60 percent.

It is difficult to predict which patients will have chronic disease, but certain factors—such as race (African-Americans are at higher risk), onset of the illness after age forty, and involvement of more than three organs—suggest a poorer prognosis.

In patients with severe involvement of the eye (loss of vision), nervous system (nerve paralysis), and heart (irregular heartbeat), the decision to administer treatment is less difficult; immediate treatment is advisable. Those patients with extensive interstitial lung involvement that may progress to fibrosis are also good candidates for immediate treatment. In some patients, severe shortness of breath combined with abnormal pulmonary function tests may also prompt early treatment.

In patients who do not have severe involvement with sarcoidosis, an observation of the course of the disease during a six-month period is advisable. Research suggests that approximately 40 percent of these patients will experience spontaneous improvement.

KYPHOSCOLIOSIS

The air sacs of the lung may be affected by diseases of the surrounding chest wall. The part of the spinal column that supports the chest is called the thoracic spine. In the normal spine, the neck has a forward curve (lordosis), whereas the thoracic spine curves backward (kyphosis). Twelve ribs surround each lung, extending in a semicircle from the spine in the back, and attaching to the breastbone (sternum) in the front. A number of diseases of the chest wall and spine can produce lung disease, as well as respiratory failure. One important example is kyphoscoliosis.

Scoliosis (crookedness) is the curvature of the spine to the side (right or left). (Actually, two curves are seen, a major curve in one direction and a smaller, compensatory curve in the opposite direction.) Scoliosis may be a birth defect or it may be acquired through disease (for example, poliomyelitis, cerebral palsy, muscular dystrophy). The normal kyphosis, or backward, convex curvature of the spine, may become increased, and individuals with this deformity are commonly called humpback or hunchbacked. These two deformities frequently coexist and are called kyphoscoliosis.

Scoliosis

In most cases, the cause of scoliosis is unknown. Scoliosis may be noted between birth (infantile) and three years of age; between ages four and ten (juvenile); and between the ages of ten and thirteen (adolescent). The earlier a child develops scoliosis, the more likely the curve will increase with the adolescent growth spurt.

Congenital scoliosis reduces the space for lung growth after birth. The infant's lungs mold themselves to the abnormal shape of the chest cavity. This restricts the growth and function of the alveoli, resulting in lowered oxygen levels. As the patient ages, the air sacs may collapse, atrophy, and become scarred or fibrotic. If not corrected, the low oxygen levels increase the pressure in the pulmonary vessels, which results in heart enlargement.

Carbon dioxide levels tend to increase with age in cases of severe scoliosis. Pneumonia and recurrent bronchial infections are common in patients with severe degrees of curvature. For these reasons, congenital spinal deformities are treated surgically to reduce curvature. This procedure should be done at an early age to avoid atrophy of the air sacs. Surgery for congenital scoliosis after age twenty-five rarely improves lung function.

Scoliosis may increase in adults after full maturity, producing pain and disability as they age. This is much more likely in patients with larger curves and those who are sedentary and overweight. Progression is also commonly seen in women with scoliosis at menopause, especially when osteoporosis is present.

Kyphosis

The most common form of kyphosis of the thoracic spine occurs due to poor posture (round-shouldered). This problem usually begins in adolescence and is more common in girls who are self-conscious about breast development. Postural exercises and occasional bracing may be necessary to correct this problem.

Like scoliosis, kyphosis may be a congenital birth defect. This deformity may cause nerve weakness or paralysis and frequently requires surgical correction.

SYMPTOMS OF KYPHOSCOLIOSIS

The most common symptom of patients with kyphoscoliosis is shortness of breath. In general, the greater the curvature, the greater the incidence of pulmonary symptoms. Repeated infections in these patients may lead to bronchiectasis or chronic bronchitis. In these patients, cough and sputum production may be frequent complaints.

PULMONARY FUNCTION TESTS IN KYPHOSCOLIOSIS

Patients with moderate to severe kyphoscoliosis have small lung volumes on pulmonary function testing. Airflows in these patients are normal unless they have smoked or experienced recurrent bronchitis. In patients with severe curvature, blood gases reveal low oxygen and high carbon dioxide levels.

TREATMENT OF SCOLIOSIS

The best treatment for scoliosis is early detection. Scoliosis screening is performed in the United States, usually in the fifth grade (ages ten to eleven years). If detected early, most curves can be treated without surgery. Treatment should be directed at a scoliosis center and may involve an exercise program and bracing.

Surgery for scoliosis involves fusing the bony units of the spine to stabilize and correct the curve. Surgery is required for progressive curvature of the spine despite bracing, as well as for loss of lung function. It may also be done to relieve pain and for cosmetic changes in the shoulders and trunk.

Don't Forget to Treat Osteoporosis

Osteoporosis is a bone condition that often leads to crippling spine and hip fractures and commonly exacerbates kyphoscoliosis. At least half of all postmenopausal women and up to one-fifth of men older than age seventy are affected by osteoporosis.

Bone is constantly being broken down (resorbed) and rebuilt. With age, more bone is resorbed than is replaced. In women, the process is accelerated around menopause because of a decline of estrogen. Osteoporosis occurs when the resorption causes the bone to reach a fracture threshold—the point at which bones are likely to break when subjected to mild stress, such as coughing. The signs of osteoporosis, such as back pain, stooped posture, and loss of height, usually occur within five years of reaching the fracture threshold.

When osteoporosis occurs in the thoracic spine, it produces fractures of the vertebrae, creating increased kyphosis. In patients with preexisting curvature, the added curve exacerbates the condition and produces increased pain and shortness of breath from further reduction of lung capacity.

The best treatment of osteoporosis is prevention. This begins with adopting a lifestyle and diet that promote bone health. Exercise, such as walking and using light weights, should be performed regularly and patients should avoid smoking and excessive use of alcohol and caffeine. At least 1,500 milligrams of calcium and 800 international units of vitamin D should be consumed daily, either through diet or supplements. Postmenopausal women should receive hormone replacement (estrogen) unless there is a medical contraindication.

Drug therapy for osteoporosis has improved recently. Two nonhormonal agents, alendronate (Fosamax) and calcitonin nasal spray (Miacalcin), provide additional options for treatment.

Treating the Pulmonary Complications

Kyphoscoliosis impacts breathing by greatly increasing the work of the respiratory muscles. Patients with severe curvature and fatigue of these muscles often present with respiratory failure, which is manifested by low oxygen and high carbon dioxide levels. The carbon dioxide levels have been seen to increase further during sleep. Signs of heart failure, such as swelling, as well as cyanosis are common in these patients.

In these patients with respiratory failure, assisted respiration is necessary. Artificial respirators deliver a specified amount of air and oxygen to the lungs and increase the excretion of carbon dioxide. In the patient with respiratory failure and kyphoscoliosis, the most beneficial approach is to deliver the "extra breaths" from a respirator through a small mask that fits over the nasal passages. In many patients, this device can be used exclusively at night, when the abnormalities in blood gases are more severe. Prolonged use of this assisted respiration allows the fatigued respiratory muscles to regain their strength so that the patient can ultimately resume normal activities during the day.

Patients with kyphoscoliosis who also develop airway disease, such as bronchitis or emphysema, will benefit from bronchodilator therapy. Many patients with severe kyphoscoliosis develop bronchiectasis after repeated bouts of pneumonia. Physical therapy, including postural drainage, is important to help mobilize secretions from clogged bronchial tubes in these patients.

ADDING TO THE LIST OF LUNG DISEASES

Diseases that affect the air sacs of the lung seem to increase almost daily. Interstitial lung diseases are often produced by exposure to an offending substance at work or in the home. As noted in this chapter, a device as simple as a humidifier may produce interstitial lung disease. Increased awareness of this form of lung disorder, as well as proper regulation of occupations at risk for these diseases will hopefully reduce the number of cases.

The lung's air sacs may also be affected by many other chest disorders. Kyphoscoliosis is only one example of a chest disease in which the alveoli are compressed and collapsed. Unfortunately, the scope of this book cannot include the vast number of infections that may attack the alveoli. Information on infectious diseases of the lung, however, may be found in the appendix.

In the preceding two chapters, diseases of the bronchial tubes and air sacs have been discussed. A vast network of blood vessels also exists within the lungs. Diseases that affect these vital channels are discussed in the next chapter.

5

DISEASES OF THE PULMONARY VESSELS

The blood vessels of the lungs must accommodate the body's entire supply of blood to facilitate the exchange of oxygen and carbon dioxide in the alveoli. The lung blood vessels are thin walled, allowing sudden increases in blood flow, which may occur during exercise, for example. The pressure in these blood channels is low in comparison to that in the general circulation. If the pressure in the pulmonary vessels rises (pulmonary hypertension), it is transmitted through the vessels to the chambers of the right side of the heart. Sustained elevation of pressure within the pulmonary vessels may then cause the right ventricle to enlarge (cor pulmonale) and ultimately fail. Many breathing and total-body disorders affect the pulmonary vessels. This chapter discusses two of these disorders: primary pulmonary hypertension and pulmonary emboli.

PRIMARY PULMONARY HYPERTENSION

Primary pulmonary hypertension (PPH) is a condition of unknown cause in which the pulmonary vessels become progressively narrowed and obstructed. This blockage produces huge increases in pressure in the vessels, which may result in heart failure.

Several behaviors have been associated with PPH, including the ingestion of appetite suppressants. Among the agents that may produce PPH are fenfluramine (Pondamin) and dexfenfluramine (Redux), both of which were withdrawn by the FDA in 1997. Fenfluramine combined with phentermine (Fastin, Adipex-P) formed the popular Fen-Phen treatment for obesity.

Many other substances have been associated with the development of PPH, including extracts from the *Papilionaceae crotalaria* plant species, which are used in parts of Africa and the Caribbean to make herbal tea. Patients ingesting rapeseed oil and L-tryptophan have also been found to develop pulmonary hypertension.

PPH occurs twice as frequently in women as in men. The disease is most common between the ages of twenty and fifty but may occur at any age. PPH may occasionally occur in families, suggesting that it may be transmitted genetically.

Symptoms of PPH

The most common symptom of PPH is shortness of breath noted on exertion. Patients may also complain of fatigue and chest pain or pressure. Fainting spells (syncope) are also common in pulmonary hypertension. Patients with advanced disease may also complain of leg swelling. In approximately 30 percent of patients, the blood vessels of the hands constrict, producing blanching of the skin, and pain (Raynaud's phenomenon).

Signs of PPH

The physical findings of PPH are related to the effect of the increase in pressure within the lung's blood vessels. The increased turbulence of blood flow and pressure within the large pulmonary vessels commonly produces a change in the heart sounds, which the physician may detect with a stethoscope. A heart murmur and alteration in the sounds related to blood flow into the pulmonary vessels may also be noted. Evidence of heart failure, such as swollen neck veins and swelling of the liver and legs, may be noted in advanced cases of PPH.

How Is PPH Diagnosed?

PPH is diagnosed by identifying the features of this disease and by excluding all known causes of pulmonary hypertension. The physician begins with the plain chest x-ray, which typically reveals enlargement of the pulmonary arteries. Enlargement of the chambers of the right side of the heart may also be noted. A chest CAT scan and MRI are also helpful in excluding other causes of pulmonary hypertension, such as emphysema and interstitial fibrosis.

Another technique used in the diagnosis of diseases of the pulmonary vessels involves the injection of a nuclear tracer substance (perfusion lung scan). Once injected, the lungs are scanned to see the distribution of the radioactive tracer. If a blood vessel is blocked, the tracer cannot enter and a "defect" is seen in the scan. This technique is also performed after the patient inhales a radioactive substance (ventilation lung scan). By comparing the perfusion and ventilation studies, the physician is better able to determine the source of a defect. Patients with PPH have a characteristic pattern on lung scanning.

A routine electrocardiogram often reflects the enlargement of the chambers of the right side of the heart. Echocardiography is helpful in excluding structural heart problems, diseases of the heart valves, for example, which may also cause pulmonary hypertension. The echocardiogram has also been used to detect elevated pulmonary artery pressures.

In a patient suspected of having PPH, a more detailed examination of heart function (cardiac catheterization) is usually required. This technique allows direct measurement of pressures in the pulmonary vessels, as well as within the chambers of the heart.

IS A BIOPSY NECESSARY?

The use of open-lung biopsy in the diagnosis of PPH is controversial because the diagnosis can usually be made based on the above findings. In patients suspected of having another form of pulmonary hypertension, open lung biopsy may be necessary because the treatment of other disorders may be different.

Treatment of PPH

MEDICAL THERAPY

In PPH, the blood vessels of the lungs are narrowed or constricted. This disease's primary treatment is the administration of a group of medications that open or dilate the blood vessels (vasodilators). One of these medications, prostacyclin, is administered through a vein and is considered the drug of choice for the treatment of PPH. Vasodilators reduce pressure within the pulmonary vessels. This results in improvement in the action of the heart in approximately 25 percent of patients with PPH. In the remaining patients, vasodilator therapy may produce only mild improvement or adversely affect the disease. Adverse reactions appear more often in patients with heart failure.

SURGICAL THERAPY: TRANSPLANTATION

Patients with PPH and heart failure usually succumb to their disease within one to two years. Patients with milder symptoms and better heart function survive longer but still have a poor outlook. Due to this poor prognosis, combined heart-lung transplantation has been considered the treatment of choice for patients who have not responded to medical therapy. A lack of organ donors, however, has limited this procedure's availability. The average time on a waiting list for combined heart-lung transplantation and single lung transplant is eighteen to twenty-four months and twelve to eighteen months, respectively.

Transplantation is, of course, not without significant risks. Post-transplant patients may suffer organ rejection and experience infections due to the use of antirejection drugs that lower immune defenses.

PULMONARY EMBOLISM

In the United States, more than 630,000 people experience pulmonary embolism each year. This disorder is the primary cause of death in 100,000 individuals annually and a contributing cause of death in another 100,000 patients. More than half of these deaths occur in patients in whom the diagnosis of pulmonary embolism is never made. Death from pulmonary embolism may be sudden, with more than 60,000 individuals dying within the first hour of the event.

Why Is It So Hard to Detect?

Pulmonary embolism is difficult to diagnosis because no symptom, sign, or routine laboratory test is specific to this disorder. Other lung diseases may mask the findings of pulmonary embolism, preventing or delaying diagnosis. Since early diagnosis and treatment greatly improve survival, the physician must have a high index of suspicion for this disease. At times, treatment must be initiated before a definite diagnosis has been made.

What Is an Embolus?

Oxygen-rich blood is pumped by the heart into vessels, called arteries, which circulate throughout the body. Vessels, called veins, return the oxygen-depleted blood to the lungs for new gas exchange. A blood clot (thrombus) may form in a vein and be dislodged and carried in the bloodstream (embolus). When such a clot enters the lung it is called a pulmonary embolus and the event is called a pulmonary embolism.

Where Does the Clot Form?

A blood clot may form in any vein in the body but is most commonly found in the leg's veins. Blood naturally collects in the veins of the lower limbs due to gravity. As the muscles of the legs contract, blood is pushed upward toward larger vessels that lead to the heart and lungs. The veins of the leg have thin walls, which may expand and become tortuous over time and are called varicose. Varicose veins are more likely to develop clots due to a decrease in blood flow. When a clot forms, inflammation develops, and the condition is called phlebitis. Venous thrombophlebitis is the medical term commonly used to describe the formation of blood clots within a vein. If this clot breaks off and travels in the body's circulation, it is called a venous thromboembolism.

Why Does the Clot Form?

Several factors have been implicated in the development of blood clots (thrombi), including decreased blood flow, trauma to the vessel, and accelerated clotting.

When blood stagnates in a vessel, there is a greater risk of clotting. One of the most common situations in which pulmonary emboli occur is following a long trip during which the patient has been sitting in one position for several hours.

When a blood vessel is injured, as in a fall or from surgery, a clot may form at the site. Some injuries are treated with a cast or splint to immobilize the limb. This decreases flow through the injured vessel. Patients after surgery are often required to stay in bed, increasing stagnation of blood and increasing the risk of clot formation.

The blood contains many elements that promote clotting. An imbalance in these elements or clotting factors may produce accelerated clotting, which leads to the formation of thrombi.

Table 5.1 lists a number of factors that are known to increase the risk of clotting and embolism. One of the most common is the use of oral contraceptives, which increase the risk of thromboembolism sixfold. The development of venous thrombi is also associated with several malignancies, such as cancer of the pancreas and lung. In some of these patients, the development of thrombi may be the first sign of malignancy.

Symptoms of Pulmonary Embolism

The most common symptom of pulmonary embolism is the sudden onset of shortness of breath. This presentation contrasts sharply with that of many of the chronic lung diseases discussed previously, where breathlessness occurs gradually. In patients with pulmonary embolism, air hunger may occur at rest.

TABLE 5.1 RISK FACTORS FOR DEVELOPING CLOT AND EMBOLISM

1. Prior episodes of clotting and embolism

2. Heart disease, such as congestive heart failure and irregular heart rhythms

3. Cancer

4. Major surgery

5. Injuries to the legs, hips, and pelvis

6. Pregnancy

7. Estrogen therapy: hormone replacement or oral contraceptives

8. Immobilization or paralysis

9. Overactive clotting

When a blood clot impacts the pulmonary blood vessels it fragments almost immediately. The smaller clots travel farther into the blood vessels. When the clot finally lodges in a smaller vessel it causes a local reaction. Since the smaller blood vessels are located near the outer surface membrane of the lung (pleura), the lodged clot may irritate the pleura. This irritation causes pain felt upon inhalation, coughing, or sneezing, and is called pleuritic chest pain.

Cough is another common symptom of pulmonary embolism, and 30 percent of patients expectorate blood (hemoptysis). In patients with massive blood clots, fainting (syncope) is common. A massive clot may effectively block the main pulmonary vessels and place severe strain on the heart.

Pulmonary embolism may occur silently. These clots are smaller and may therefore not produce symptoms. In these patients, shortness of breath occurs gradually and the disease state may resemble PPH.

Signs of Pulmonary Embolism

A rapid rate of breathing (tachypnea) is the most common finding in patients after pulmonary embolism has occurred. A rapid heart rate (tachycardia) is found in 40 percent of patients. Fever may also occur but is usually not greater than 101 degrees Fahrenheit. The chest sounds are also not specific to this disease. In a small percentage of patients, wheezing is audible. In the patient with pleural reaction to the pulmonary embolus, a leathery sound, called a friction rub, may be heard. Unfortunately, this finding is often fleeting and may not be recognized when it occurs.

LABORATORY FINDINGS:
HOW THE DIAGNOSIS IS MADE

Blood Testing
No specific blood test exists for the diagnosis of pulmonary embolism. Many patients with pulmonary embolism, however, have changes in the

blood, which reflect the breakdown of blood clots. Further development of this type of blood analysis may yet yield a helpful marker for this disease.

Blood-Gas Analysis

The exchange of oxygen and carbon dioxide in the alveolar sacs may be affected by pulmonary emboli. Small clots, however, may not produce any significant changes. In patients with larger clots or repeated episodes, blood oxygen levels fall. Due to the rapid breathing rate, patients may excrete more carbon dioxide and have low CO_2 levels.

Chest X-Ray

Chest x-rays of patients with pulmonary emboli are primarily useful for eliminating other chest diseases but are not specific for diagnosis. A normal chest x-ray is common, especially with smaller blood clots. Larger emboli may produce a variety of abnormalities that reflect bleeding within or collapse of air sacs (atelectasis). In patients with pleural reaction, there may be signs of fluid within the chest cavity (pleural effusion).

Lung Scanning: Noninvasive Diagnosis

A lung scan may provide sufficient evidence for the diagnosis of pulmonary embolism. A diagnostic scan reveals significant defects in blood flow (perfusion) with normal air exchange (ventilation) in the affected areas. A normal perfusion scan almost eliminates the diagnosis and may point the physician toward an alternative diagnosis.

Pulmonary Angiogram: Invasive but Necessary

In many patients, the results of lung scanning are equivocal and the diagnosis of pulmonary embolism can only be made by performing a pulmonary angiogram. In this technique, dye is injected into the pulmonary vessels, which allows the physician to directly visualize blocked or partially obstructed blood vessels.

Pulmonary angiography is the most accurate technique for the diagnosis of pulmonary embolism, but it is also the most invasive. Serious complications occur in less than 2 percent of patients undergoing this procedure, and approximately one out of a thousand patients will die as a consequence of this procedure alone. Patients who suffer serious complications are typically those with massive emboli or severe underlying heart and lung disease.

Treatment of Pulmonary Embolism: Anticoagulation

Once pulmonary embolism has occurred, the focus of treatment is to thin the patient's blood to prevent further clots. This process is called anticoagulation and the drug of choice is a medication known as heparin, which acts by altering a major clotting factor in the blood so that further clots do not form and emboli do not recur. This medication is usually given intravenously but may also be injected under the skin (subcutaneously). Heparin is typically given for five to ten days, after which a second drug called warfarin (Coumadin), which can be taken by mouth, continues the process of anticoagulation. Coumadin works much more slowly than heparin and requires days to achieve its effect. Its primary action is to reduce the production of clotting factors in the liver.

The most important and striking adverse effect of both heparin and Coumadin is bleeding. If the blood becomes too thin or if the patient has another problem, such as a stomach ulcer, hemorrhage may occur; this can be life threatening. For this reason, patients receiving anticoagulants must have their blood strictly monitored to determine the magnitude of the effect of these drugs.

Alternative Treatment

Heparin and Coumadin do not break up (lyse) the blood clot. Thrombolytic therapy acts directly to dissolve clots. Three thrombolytic agents, streptokinase, urokinase, and tissue plasminogen activator

(TPA), are available for the treatment of blood clots. Like anticoagulants, the primary risk of using these agents is bleeding and possible hemorrhage.

Thrombolytic therapy is only used in patients with massive pulmonary emboli and who do not respond to anticoagulation within the first twenty-four to forty-eight hours. These patients have usually developed heart strain or failure and may be in shock when they are first seen.

Can the Clots Be Removed?

Surgery to remove blood clots in the pulmonary vessels can be performed in patients who fail to respond to medical therapy. Patients who undergo embolectomy typically have had massive blood clots and have developed heart failure. The procedure carries with it significant risk, especially if pulmonary hypertension has developed.

Better Than Treatment: Prevention

Pulmonary emboli occur as a consequence of the formation of blood clots in another site, usually a leg vein. This disorder may be prevented entirely if the distant clot does not form or is treated promptly, before it can travel through the circulation.

For this reason, prophylactic measures are taken in the high-risk group of patients noted in the preceding discussion. These include beginning anticoagulation when a patient becomes immobilized or has surgery. Compression stockings to improve the return of blood from the veins of the legs are commonly used. Devices that actually compress the legs with air are also now used in selected patients.

Patients who have had episodes of venous thrombosis or pulmonary emboli are treated with blood thinners for an extended period of time. In those individuals who have had repeated episodes, this form of treatment may be continued for life. Many patients are advised to wear compression stockings and to avoid prolonged periods of sitting.

TAKING CONTROL OF YOUR DISEASE

The last three chapters have described many types of breathing disorders. These disorders may produce severe breathlessness, resulting in a marked change in the ability of the affected individual to work and continue an active and full life. Air hunger often affects the mind, as well as the body, producing fear that further restricts activity. The next chapter discusses methods that allow patients with chest disease to resume control of their lives.

6

PULMONARY REHABILITATION

Once the diagnosis of a chronic breathing disorder, such as emphysema, chronic bronchitis, asthma, or interstitial lung disease, has been made, many patients will benefit from a program of pulmonary rehabilitation. This is designed to improve the quality of life and increase the ability of individuals with these disorders to function at their highest capacity.

Patients with chronic lung diseases frequently have had to stop working and may have become homebound, unable to perform simple chores or enjoy activities that require even light exertion. For some, the act of getting dressed each morning may have become nearly impossible ("I can't even put on my pants!"). This constant struggle for breath typically produces anxiety and depression, which further act to restrict the patient's activities.

Pulmonary rehabilitation programs utilize a team approach of physician, nurse specialist, physical therapist, dietitian, social worker, and psychologist working with the patient. Many medical centers now offer a program that combines education, exercise, and nutritional and psychological counseling.

This chapter outlines some of the material that is offered in rehabilitation programs. It is not intended as a substitute for enrolling in a formal program but is an introduction to the process of pulmonary rehabilitation. For many, pulmonary rehabilitation is the first step toward resuming normal activities.

BREATHING EXERCISES

As noted, many of the chronic lung diseases that have been discussed produce severe air hunger and a rapid rate of breathing. Patients with these diseases tend to take many small breaths each minute. When sustained, this pattern of breathing produces fatigue of the respiratory muscles, and these fatigued muscles frequently precedes respiratory failure.

When these patients are observed, it is often obvious that they are breathing with their chest muscles and not with the diaphragm and abdominal muscles. As discussed below, abdominal, or "belly breathing," is the more natural and effective method of breathing.

Which Are the Respiratory Muscles?

Many muscles support respiration and may become fatigued from lung disorders that produce increased work of breathing. The primary muscles of breathing are the diaphragm and the muscles between each of the ribs. The diaphragm is responsible for 75 percent of the effort of breathing. The belly, or abdominal muscles, are also important in breathing and assist the chest structures. The abdominal muscles girdle the front of the belly.

Recent research has also demonstrated that the muscles of the neck (often called "strap muscles") that attach to the chest and upper arms also assist in breathing. These muscles are often easily seen when an individual develops severe shortness of breath. They are often called "accessory muscles" of breathing.

The intercostal and accessory muscles are relatively small and are quickly fatigued by an increase in the work of breathing. Patients who overwork these muscles are prone to respiratory failure.

Specific Exercises

Several simple breathing exercises may help reduce shortness of breath. The goal of these exercises is to change the patient's breathing pattern from the rapid, small breaths described above to a slower, deeper, more relaxed pattern of breathing. Through practice, many patients can achieve this change and reduce air hunger. There is no substitute for a good teacher, and these exercises are best introduced by an experienced professional.

PURSED-LIP BREATHING

Pursed-lip breathing is useful in the COPD patient. In COPD, air passages close prematurely, trapping air in the lungs. Air goes in but does not come out, creating large, overinflated lungs. The air that is trapped in the lungs in COPD is not used for exchange of oxygen or carbon dioxide and simply takes up space. Pursed-lip breathing attempts to remove the stale air from the lungs by keeping the air passages open longer.

Performing Pursed-Lip Breathing

1. Inhale through your nose a normal amount of air while keeping your mouth closed.
2. Exhale slowly through your mouth with your lips in the whistling position (pursed).
3. Allow twice as long to exhale as to inhale. It may be helpful to count while you do this. For example, count 1, 2, slowly as you inhale and 1, 2, 3, 4, as you exhale.
4. Practice pursed-lip breathing first while lying down, sitting, standing, and finally while walking so that it becomes your normal pattern of breathing.
5. When an attack of breathlessness occurs, begin to purse-lip breathe. It will slow your breathing rate and produce a more relaxed, satisfying breath. Many of my patients can demonstrate that they are able to increase their oxygen levels by pursed-lip breathing. Try it, it works.

ABDOMINAL (DIAPHRAGMATIC) BREATHING

Abdominal or diaphragmatic is the natural mode of breathing. Individuals with lung disease frequently depart from the normal pattern, overusing the chest and accessory muscles for breathing. Abdominal breathing may be used by any patient with lung disease, including asthma. Many people with normal lungs do not breathe correctly and may benefit from learning abdominal, or belly breathing.

In normal breathing with inspiration, the diaphragm moves downward toward the abdomen. This creates an outward swelling of the belly and expands the chest, allowing air to fill the lungs. At the same time, the lower ribs expand, as do the muscles in the lower back, creating more space for lung expansion. The greater filling of the lungs produces a higher oxygen level in the blood and slows the heart rate. Abdominal breathing also stimulates the parasympathetic nervous system, producing feelings of calm and relaxation. This explains why abdominal breathing is an integral part of many spiritual disciplines, such as yoga.

How to Belly Breathe

1. Abdominal breathing can be performed in any position, but it is best to start by lying on your back with your knees bent. Place your right hand on your belly just below the lower ribs.

2. Now breathe into your hand so that you can feel and see your abdomen and hand rise with inspiration. Do this slowly, and exhale. Try to clear your mind and focus on your breathing.

3. After practicing abdominal breathing on your back, turn to each side and perform the same maneuver. Now try combining pursed-lip breathing with this abdominal exercise.

4. The next step is to repeat the exercise in the sitting position. Avoid stooping over, which compresses the lungs. Try to relax your neck and shoulder muscles. In the sitting position, it may be helpful to place your other hand on your chest. Try to breathe in only from the abdomen as your chest (and other hand) stay still. When you have mastered the maneuver while sitting, move on to standing and then to walking.

5. Try to make abdominal breathing your normal pattern for each and every breath—not only for a few minutes each day.

CONDITIONING EXERCISES

One of the most damaging results of lung disease and the sensation of shortness of breath is inactivity. For many patients, routine activities, such as getting dressed or taking a shower, become overwhelmingly fatiguing. The unpleasantness of air hunger also produces significant psychological effects. Patients fear the sensation of breathlessness and avoid any form of exertion, especially walking. Unfortunately, the lack of exercise further weakens the muscles that support breathing and exacerbates the underlying breathing disorder. Instead of avoiding breathlessness, the deconditioned individual experiences even greater distress with movement.

Only through regular exercise can this process be reversed and shortness of breath decreased. Each patient should consult with a physician before starting any exercise program. A formal exercise or stress test may be necessary. A formal rehabilitation program is preferred because it allows appropriate observation during exercise.

Some General Rules

1. Establish a routine so that you exercise at the same time, preferably on a daily basis. Schedule your daily exercise session the way you would schedule an important appointment, and keep it.
2. Don't exercise if you have a cold or any infection that has decreased your energy level.
3. Stop exercising if you feel dizzy, nauseous, faint, short of breath, or develop chest pain or unusual discomfort. You should report any of these symptoms to your physician.
4. Avoid exercising outdoors during extremes of weather or on high-pollution days. Allergic patients should also check pollen counts.

How to Get Started: Warm-Up

Every exercise program should start with warm-up exercises, which are best performed while sitting. It is best to combine upper- and lower-body exercises during this warm-up period. For the lower limbs try marching while sitting or extending the knees (alternate legs). A useful upper-body warm-up exercise is as follows:

1. While sitting, place your hands at your chest with your elbows up.
2. Breathe in through your nose while extending your arms to either side.
3. Breathe out slowly through pursed lips while bringing your arms back to the original position.
4. Repeat ten times.

Walking Is the Best Exercise

The most beneficial exercise is walking. Your goal should be a twelve-minute walk without stopping. A rest period or periods are acceptable, especially when getting started. As your body becomes conditioned, you will notice that you require fewer rest periods. It is best to begin on a flat surface. A treadmill may be useful but is not essential. After achieving the goal of a twelve-minute walk without stopping, begin to lengthen the time until you have reached thirty minutes.

HOW FAST SHOULD I GO?

An exact prescription for exercise can be made from a preliminary exercise test performed by your physician. This testing is usually performed on the treadmill so that the physician can use the results as a guide for training. An exercise test will also establish if oxygen should be offered during exercise. In many patients with COPD and pulmonary fibrosis, oxygen levels may drop during exercise. Exercise testing before beginning an exercise program is highly recommended and is incorporated in pulmonary rehabilitation programs.

If an exercise test has not been done, it is best for the patient to walk at a comfortable pace that produces a moderate degree of breathlessness. Patients should avoid any exercise that produces severe shortness of breath, which may be defined as a level of breathlessness that prevents speech. It is helpful to set goals and to gradually increase exercise time.

What Other Exercises Should I Do?

In addition to walking to develop body conditioning, several other exercises may be performed. Much attention has been focused on strengthening the muscles of the upper body to assist the chest muscles. One of these exercises is described on page 182. Light weights may be used for these exercises. You do not need any special equipment. My patients use cans of soup or tomato paste for these exercises. The number of repetitions of these exercises can be fewer than suggested and gradually increased. (See the appendix for information on more exercises.)

To Strengthen the Upper Body

1. In the sitting position, place your hands on your shoulders.
2. Breathe in through your nose as you raise your arms toward the ceiling.
3. Exhale slowly through pursed lips as you return your hands to your shoulders.
4. Repeat ten times.
5. Perform the same maneuver holding one-pound weights (may increase).
6. Repeat five times.

Cooling Down

Exercise sessions should never end abruptly. It is advisable to slowly reduce exercise so that your breathing rate gradually decreases to your normal level.

POSTURAL DRAINAGE: A MUST FOR BRONCHIECTASIS

Many chronic lung conditions produce an excessive amount of secretion in the air passages of the lungs. One of the most striking examples of this increased mucus production is in bronchiectasis. Many patients with chronic bronchitis also have a buildup of mucus and clogged bronchial tubes. The clearance of this excess mucus is essential if patients are to avoid repeated infection. The drainage of mucus also decreases shortness of breath.

What Is Postural Drainage?

Postural drainage is the positioning of patients to allow gravity to assist the flow (and subsequent expectoration) of bronchial mucus. With proper positioning, each lobe of the lungs can be drained by this passive process. Each position is held for five to ten minutes or longer, depending on the individual. In many patients with bronchiectasis, a specific lobe has been damaged and postural drainage can be focused on this area.

WHO SHOULD PERFORM POSTURAL DRAINAGE?

A licensed chest physical therapist should introduce postural drainage to the patient. The therapist receives from the physician a prescription that should specify the diagnosis, as well as which lobes require drainage. In many cases, the patient can be taught the proper positioning. At home, postural drainage may be combined with routine activities, such as reading.

ADDING PERCUSSION TO POSTURAL DRAINAGE

Postural drainage is a purely passive process. To assist the drainage of mucus, percussion of the chest is performed while the patient is positioned for postural drainage. Percussion is the rhythmic clapping of the chest by a therapist or caregiver. The force applied to the chest is transmitted to the underlying lung and loosens bronchial secretion.

The technique of chest percussion requires training. The therapist's hands are cupped and apply a certain amount of force to specific areas. Many patients find the rhythm of percussion relaxing and comforting. In many instances, with proper instruction and supervision a family member can be taught to apply percussion. Some patients become adept at using one of their hands for self-percussion. Pneumatic, mechanical devices are also available; they may be applied to the chest to produce percussion and facilitate drainage of bronchial mucus.

ADDING VIBRATION AND SHAKING
TO POSTURAL DRAINAGE

Two other techniques that are used to actively loosen secretion during postural drainage are vibration and shaking. Both are performed to help move secretion from the outer, smaller bronchial tubes to the larger bronchi, where they may be expectorated.

In vibration, tension is produced in the therapist's arms and shoulders and is transmitted to the patient's chest (and lungs) through the hands. Vibration is usually performed after percussion.

Shaking is a more active process in which a bouncing motion is applied to the patient's chest. Many therapists alternate percussion with shaking to help mobilize secretions.

Both of these techniques again require a trained, experienced therapist. Mechanical vibrators, however, may provide some assistance and can be applied to specified areas.

GENERAL SUGGESTIONS FOR POSTURAL DRAINAGE

1. It is always necessary for the physician to prescribe postural drainage and to ensure that it is performed by the proper individual. The therapist should discuss treatment with the physician.
2. If bronchodilator medication has been prescribed, postural drainage is best performed after its use. A home nebulizer treatment before drainage may help loosen thick secretion.
3. As a general rule, patients should drink liberally to thin bronchial secretions. It is important to check with your physician to confirm that this is permitted, because some patients with heart disease, for example, may be restricted in their fluid intake.

THE IMPORTANCE OF PROPER DIET

Proper nutrition can play an important role in the treatment of patients with chronic lung disease. Many patients with breathing disorders are undernourished, which further weakens their breathing muscles. The opposite condition of being overweight may also increase shortness of breath, because breathing disorders may also influence how and when a patient eats. In COPD patients, for example, eating a large meal may increase breathlessness.

The Ideal Weight

Your ideal weight is based on your height, age, and sex. Tables of normal weights are available from your physician or nutritionist and may also be found in many references. (See the appendix.) Energy intake also varies from person to person, depending on age, sex, and physical activity. Sedentary women and older adults require about sixteen hundred calories a day, while active women and sedentary men require two thousand calories. These values are for normal adults. If the energy intake does not meet the body's needs, weight loss occurs, and fat and protein stored in the body is used to supply the energy needed.

Nutrients are classified into five major groups: proteins, carbohydrates, fats, vitamins, and minerals. These groups are essential for maintaining normal growth and health. Foods can roughly be classified into breads and cereals, vegetables and fruits, meat, fish, eggs, milk and milk products, fats and oils, and sugars. Vegetables and fruits are a direct source of many minerals and vitamins. Meat, fish, and eggs supply the building blocks of protein, called amino acids. Milk and dairy products also supply protein, phosphorus, calcium, and vitamins. Fats, oils, and sugars are high in calories but usually contain few nutrients.

As a general rule, you should eat a variety of foods, maintain your ideal weight, and avoid too much fat, cholesterol, sugar, and salt.

WHAT'S WRONG WITH BEING THIN?

Patients with emphysema tend to be underweight. In many, the loss of weight may resemble the wasting that is found in cancer. Numerous patients have been referred to me for evaluation for malignancy, when, in fact, the cause was emphysema. These patients usually have a great deal of muscle wasting and look emaciated.

The source of weight loss from emphysema is a combination of increased use of calories for breathing and a poor diet. In emphysema, a great deal of energy is expended for breathing. This increased work of breathing requires a large number of calories, which might normally be conserved and result in weight gain. Patients with emphysema tend to have poor appetites, partly because of increased shortness of breath that is noted after eating. Many individuals fear this sensation and choose not to eat.

The result of a poor diet is wasting of muscle, including the respiratory muscles that support breathing. This results in weakening of the breathing apparatus, which results in increased shortness of breath. This vicious cycle may mean profound weight loss.

A diet deficient in calories, as well as protein and vitamins may also reduce immunity, resulting in respiratory infection. Repeated chest infections are common in COPD and are partly due to poor nutrition. Infection may also decrease appetite and consume calories, producing further weight loss.

BEING OVERWEIGHT INCREASES SHORTNESS OF BREATH

Many patients with chronic bronchitis are overweight. Obesity is also associated with sleep apnea (which was discussed in Chapter 4). The obese COPD patient tends to have swelling of the legs due to water retention. Excess fat in the abdomen pushes up on the diaphragm, resulting in compression of the lower lungs. The space that the lungs would normally use for expansion is lost, so the air sacs collapse. This decreased lung capacity from obesity further compromises breathing and increases breathlessness.

Obesity also increases the demands on the heart and lungs to supply oxygen to all areas of the body. When demands exceed supply and delivery of oxygen due to breathing disorders, heart failure may occur.

How to Meet Your Nutritional Needs

Whenever possible, a consultation with a nutritionist is highly recommended. Most pulmonary rehabilitation programs offer this valuable resource. A nutritionist can plan a specific dietary program, while assessing your nutritional state. The following are some general suggestions:

1. It is important to consume an adequate number of calories, even if you are trying to lose weight. Remember that your work of breathing may consume large numbers of calories. Caloric supplements, such as Ensure, Sustacal, and Carnation Instant Breakfast, provide approximately 350 calories per serving and may be helpful.

2. Protein is important for the maintenance and repair of the body's cells. A dietitian should determine the amount of protein needed in your diet. Protein levels may be affected by certain medical conditions, such as kidney or liver disease. A good general rule is to consume six ounces of protein and two cups of milk per day.

3. Individuals with breathing disorders should drink at least eight cups of caffeine-free liquid per day. This fluid thins the bronchial mucus and allows it to be cleared more easily. Patients who use oxygen therapy often complain of dryness of the nose and mouth and will benefit from drinking more fluids. However, certain medical conditions, such as heart and kidney failure, require fluid restriction. Your physician should advise you if forcing fluids is not permitted.

4. Your diet should contain adequate amounts of potassium, a key body element that is involved in muscle contraction, as well as blood-pressure control. Potassium is found in citrus fruits, bananas, vegetables, dairy, and meat. A deficiency of potassium may result in muscle weakness, as well as painful cramping. Corticosteroids and diuretics (water pills) often deplete the body of potassium.

5. Calcium is another important substance that should be included in your diet and is found in dairy products, vegetables, and supplements. This material is the building block for bone and is also involved in blood-pressure control. Corticosteroids produce loss of calcium from bone and may cause osteoporosis. (See Chapter 4.)

Women are more likely to develop osteoporosis, but this condition may also affect men.

FOR COPD PATIENTS: MORE FAT, LESS CARBOHYDRATE

In COPD patients who have elevated carbon dioxide levels, a diet low in carbohydrate and high in fat is recommended. Carbon dioxide is formed by the breakdown of carbohydrates, and an adjustment in dietary intake may help reduce CO_2 levels.

How Do I Lower Carbohydrates?

1. Avoid foods that contain added sugar, such as candy, jellies, highly sweetened cereals, pastries and desserts, and soft drinks. These foods offer little nutritional value.
2. Substitute foods that use artificial sweeteners. Use water-packed or juice-packed fruit with no added sugar.

How Do I Increase Fat?

1. Increase the amount of fat in your diet by choosing foods that are high in polyunsaturated and monounsaturated fats. These come from plant sources and do not contain cholesterol. Examples are vegetable oils such as canola, olive, corn, and safflower, soft margarine, low-cholesterol mayonnaise, and salad dressing made from vegetable oil.
2. Avoid saturated fats, which come mostly from animal sources and which are high in cholesterol. Examples are fatty meats, butter, cream, lard, and gravy.
3. Become a label-reader. Avoid animal fat and hydrogenated (solid) shortening. If you are given a choice between a product made with butter or one made with canola oil, choose the one with canola oil.
4. A high-fat, low-carbohydrate liquid supplement, such as Pulmocare, may be helpful. An eight-ounce can of this supplement provides 355 calories.

How Do I Eat When I Am Short of Breath?

Many patients with chronic lung disease experience increased breath-lessness after eating a full meal. This discomfort may contribute to poor dietary intake and further weight loss. The following suggestions should help you deal with this problem.

1. Instead of large meals, eat three small meals and three snacks a day.
2. The largest meal of the day should not be in the evening because it may exacerbate breathing problems at night.
3. Many patients with chronic lung disease suffer from reflux of stomach contents. Avoid eating for at least two hours before you lie down.
4. The act of eating may be tiring. Rest before eating, and choose foods that are easy to chew.

Why Am I So Gassy?

Many patients with breathing disorders complain bitterly about excess gas. This problem is partly due to the swallowing of air that occurs with rapid breathing. This condition is called aerophagia and may produce swelling of the stomach and intestines. The swollen stomach pushes up against the diaphragm, further restricting lung expansion. The result is increased shortness of breath.

This problem can be reduced by avoiding gas-causing vegetables and carbonated beverages. Foods that produce excess gas include apples (raw), asparagus, beans, broccoli, cabbage, cauliflower, corn, melons, onions (raw), peas, peppers, radishes, and turnips.

Many gas-reducing products are available without prescription. Most of them include simethicone, which breaks up gas bubbles. Activated charcoal capsules, which absorb gas, may also be of some benefit.

Should I Take Vitamins?

Vitamin and mineral deficiencies may exist in the malnourished patient with lung disease. When deficiencies exist, vitamin and mineral supplementation is necessary. The best way to assess these deficiencies is through proper evaluation by the physician and nutritionist. This evaluation includes measurement of blood levels of vitamin B_{12} and folic acid, electrolytes, protein, and a blood count. Excessive intake of certain vitamins and minerals can also be harmful. In general, a combination multivitamin and mineral supplement that provides 100 percent of the FDA's Recommended Dietary Allowances (RDA) is more than adequate, especially if combined with a healthy diet.

A recent report of using retinoic acid (a derivative of vitamin A) to successfully treat emphysema in rats has raised speculation that this treatment might be applicable to humans. Unfortunately, much time and research will be necessary to decide if these laboratory results can be duplicated in humans.

Antioxidant vitamins (beta carotene, vitamin C, vitamin E) have also received a great deal of attention recently. When the body's cells burn oxygen, by-products called oxygen-free radicals are formed. These free radicals can damage tissue, causing diseases such as cancer, heart disease, and arthritis. Environmental factors, such as cigarette smoke and ultraviolet light, may also cause free radicals to form. Antioxidants work as scavengers, mopping up free radicals and converting them to harmless waste products. The best source of the antioxidant vitamins is a diet that includes fruits, vegetables, and grains. To date, the taking of supplements of vitamins A, C, E, and beta carotene has not been shown to reduce the risk of cancer or heart disease. In fact, high doses of beta carotene have been shown to be harmful.

DEALING WITH YOUR EMOTIONS

Emotional disorders, such as anxiety and depression, are common in patients with breathing disorders. The sensation of shortness of breath, as well as the disabling effects of chronic lung disease frequently give rise to significant psychological problems. In many cases, the psychological problem may aggravate the underlying disease. In the patient with emphysema, for example, depression may further decrease appetite and activity.

How Should Anxiety Be Treated?

In many patients, anxiety is the product of severe breathlessness. Many individuals with breathing disorders report that they experience panic due to air hunger. Others note the same sensation if they forget to take their medication or find that their bronchodilator spray is empty. Patients with chronic lung disorders often express fear of losing the ability to function and becoming dependent on others.

These problems should be explored by the physician or a trained professional, often with involvement of the patient's family. Communicating these fears is the first step toward coping. A support group for individuals with breathing disorders and their families may also provide a useful forum for discussion of anxiety-producing problems. Psychotherapy may be advisable in some patients with severe anxiety.

Anxiety may also be treated with behavioral therapy that consists of relaxation and biofeedback. Many of the relaxation techniques involve breathing exercises that patients may incorporate into their daily workout.

SHOULD TRANQUILIZERS BE USED?

Antianxiety drugs, such as the benzodiazepines, may be effective in reducing the symptoms of anxiety in many patients. These medications, however, which include the widely prescribed drugs diazepam (Valium) and alprazolam (Xanax), produce sedation that may depress breathing in patients with chronic lung disease. This depression of the brain's breathing center may result in respiratory failure. For this reason, these medications may be contraindicated in many patients with breathing disorders.

Long-term use of the benzodiazepine drugs may also produce a physical dependence or addiction to these agents. In addition, when these medications are discontinued the return of symptoms is common.

One antianxiety agent, buspirone (Buspar), which belongs to another drug family called azapirone, is also useful in treating anxiety. This medication does not produce significant sedation and has not been found to depress breathing, or to produce drug dependence or addiction. Buspirone has a slower onset of action than the benzodiazepines and is generally regarded as a milder medication.

Facing Depression

Depression is found in many patients with chronic illnesses, and frequently in individuals with breathing disorders. Many patients express feelings of hopelessness when faced with a diagnosis of chronic lung disease. The restriction in activity due to breathlessness often adds to depression by isolating the patient from friends and families. Patients frequently stop going to social events due to self-consciousness over the use of portable oxygen. After I prescribed oxygen therapy for a patient with severe emphysema, she told me that she would "never leave my apartment again" to ensure that her neighbors would not know her condition.

NICOTINE FOR DEPRESSION?

In some patients, depression may have existed before the development of the breathing disorder. Recent investigation has demonstrated that for years many individuals have unknowingly used nicotine through cigarette smoking as an antidepressant. This may explain the tremendous difficulty in quitting smoking and also supports the use of an agent such as bupropion for smoking cessation. (See Chapter 4.) Although nicotine may have partially treated these patients' depression, they have also suffered the many damaging effects of cigarette smoking.

How to Approach Depression

In most cases, a depressed mood is noted by both the patient and physician. In some patients, however, depression may be manifested by other mood changes, such as irritability, anger, and restlessness. A psychological assessment is usually made on entry into most rehabilitation programs, with referral to the appropriate professional for treatment. As with the treatment of anxiety, support groups are another helpful option.

SHOULD ANTIDEPRESSANT DRUGS BE USED?

After the proper psychological evaluation, a decision to prescribe an antidepressant drug may be made. Many antidepressant medications are available. In the last ten to fifteen years, a family of antidepressants that affects a chemical called serotonin has been used extensively for depression. Examples include fluoxetine (Prozac), sertaline (Zoloft), and paroxetine (Paxil). In general, these agents do not adversely affect breathing and may be used in patients with chronic lung diseases.

WHY SHOULD MAO INHIBITORS BE AVOIDED?

An older family of antidepressant drugs is the monoamine oxidase (MAO) inhibitors. These agents may interact with a number of foods and medications, including the beta-agonists that are frequently used as bronchodilators in patients with asthma and COPD. MAO inhibitors should not be administered to patients receiving this form of bronchodilator.

ACHIEVING SUCCESS IN REHABILITATION

In many instances, chronic lung disease may dictate how an individual functions from the moment of awakening each morning until falling asleep at night. Through the efforts of physicians, physical therapists, nutritionists, and psychologists, pulmonary rehabilitation offers patients with chronic lung disease the opportunity to resume control over their lives.

Success in rehabilitation also depends on the individual's motivation. Studies have shown that the motivated patient who approaches rehabilitation with a positive, goal-oriented attitude achieves greater success in this endeavor.

Toward Better Breathing and Health

As noted, you can make many important contributions to achieving better breathing and general health. These include smoking cessation, avoidance of allergens and pollutants, proper diet and weight control, the performance of daily breathing exercises, and keeping a regular exercise routine. Whenever possible, consult with your physician for advice and support in making these lifestyle changes. None of these measures is simple or easy to achieve, and many attempts may be necessary before you succeed.

AVOIDING LUNG DISEASE

This book has focused on how we breathe, as well as the most common breathing disorders that may prompt an individual to consult a physician. The seemingly simple and automatic act of breathing is too often taken for granted. Breathing is, in fact, a complex and intricate act. Numerous disorders may affect the control of breathing or the lungs and supporting structures, producing shortness of breath and disability. Many lung diseases may be avoided by eliminating cigarette smoking and air pollution. Progress has been made in many areas, but with air pollution, for example, enforcement of established regulations is lacking.

The death rate from lung disease continues to rise, while the number of deaths from heart disease and cancer decline. A concerted effort that involves every individual who decides not to smoke will be needed to ensure that the incidence of fatal lung disease will also decline.

Given the proper funding, much of the effort to reduce lung disease will come from scientific research. Many of the disorders discussed in this book are labeled idiopathic because they do not have known causes. I have no doubt that the source of many of these diseases will be better defined in the near future. Science is also poised to add gene therapy to the treatment options for many lung diseases that have a genetic basis, including cystic fibrosis.

BREATH IS LIFE

Although breathing is automatic, it is also voluntary. Normal breathing is the life force that sustains us. Proper breathing techniques that promote relaxation and reduce breathlessness can be learned and mastered. In many cultures the word for breath and spirit are the same. By avoiding lung disease and practicing normal breathing, both the mind and the body may be renewed.

BIBLIOGRAPHY

Adams, F. V. *The Asthma Sourcebook*. Los Angeles: Lowell House, 1996.

Barnes, P. J., K. F. Chung, T. W. Evans, and S. G. Spiro. *Therapeutics in Respiratory Disease*. Edinburgh: Churchill Livingstone, 1994.

Berkow, R., M. H. Beers, and A. J. Fletcher, eds. *The Merck Manual of Medical Information*. Whitehouse Station: Merck & Co., 1997.

Bevelaqua, F. A. and F. V. Adams. "Pulmonary Disorders," in Eisenberg, M. G., R. L. Glueckauf, and H. H. Zaretsky, eds. *Medical Aspects of Disability* (325–341). New York: Springer, 1993.

Bone, R. C. "Asthma: New Treatments Will Improve Disease Management." *Clin Pulm Med* 2(5):249–257, 1995.

Boyd, G., A. H. Morice, J. C. Pounsford, et al. "An evaluation of salmeterol in the treatment of chronic obstructive pulmonary disease (COPD)." *EurRespir J* 10:815–821 (1997).

Brooks, S. M., J. E. Lockey, and P. Harber, eds. "Occupational Lung Diseases." *Clinics in Chest Medicine* 2(2):171–299, 1981.

Chediak, A. D. and B. P. Krieger. "Obstructive Sleep Apnea Syndrome." In *Pulmonary and Critical Care Medicine*, edited by R. C. Bone. St. Louis: Mosby, 1996.

Cooke, R. 1993. "A Deadly Gene's Big Surprise." *Newsday*, 17 August
    1993, 57.

Duyff, R. L. *American Dietetic Association's Complete Food & Nutrition
    Guide*. Minneapolis: Chronimed Publishing, 1996.

Fanburg, B. L. and L. Sicilian, eds. 1994. "Respiratory Dysfunction in
    Neuromuscular Disease." *Clinics in Chest Medicine* 15(4):
    607–761.

Farhi, D. *The Breathing Book*. New York: Henry Holt, 1996.

Fiel, S. B. "Cystic Fibrosis." In *Pulmonary and Critical Care Medicine*,
    edited by R. C. Bone. St. Louis: Mosby, 1995.

Filderman, A. E. and R. A. Matthay. "Bronchogenic Carcinoma." In
    Pulmonary and Critical Care Medicine, edited by R. C. Bone. St.
    Louis: Mosby, 1996.

Fiore, M. C., T. M. Piasecki, L. J. Baker, and S. M. Deeren. "Cigarette
    Smoking: The Leading Preventable Cause of Pulmonary Disease."
    In *Pulmonary and Critical Care Medicine*, edited by R. C. Bone.
    St. Louis: Mosby, 1997.

Frownfelter, D. and E. Dean, eds. *Principles and Practice of
    Cardiopulmonary Physical Therapy*. St. Louis: Mosby, 1996.

Fulmer, J. D. and A. A. Katzenstein. "The Interstitial Lung Diseases."
    In *Pulmonary and Critical Care Medicine*, edited by R. C. Bone.
    St. Louis: Mosby, 1996.

Guidelines for the Diagnosis and Management of Asthma. 1997.
    Washington, D.C.: U.S. Department of Health and Human
    Services (National Asthma Education Program).
    NIH Pub. No. 97-4051A.

Hyers, T. M., ed. 1984. "Pulmonary Embolism and Hypertension."
    Clinics in Chest Medicine. 5(3):385–550.

Irwin, R. S. and H. M. Hollingsworth. "The Upper Respiratory Tract." In *Pulmonary and Critical Care Medicine*, edited by R. C. Bone. St. Louis: Mosby, 1996.

Keim, H. A. and R. N. Hensinger. 1989. "Spinal Deformities: Scoliosis and Kyphosis." *Clinical Symposia* 41(4):3–32.

Kryger, M. H. 1983. "Sleep Apnea." *Arch Intern Med* 143:2301–2303.

———. 1985. "Fat, Sleep, and Charles Dickens." *Clinics in Chest Medicine* 6(4):555–561.

Lam, W. K. 1996. "Chemotherapy for Advanced Non–Small Cell Lung Cancer." *Clin Pulm Med* 3(5):288–292.

Lung Disease Data 1997. New York: American Lung Association, 1997.

Newman, L. S., C. S. Rose, and L. A. Maier. 1997 "Sarcoidosis." *The New England Journal of Medicine* 336:1224–1234.

Owens, G. R. "Chronic Obstructive Pulmonary Disease." In *Pulmonary and Critical Care Medicine*, edited by R. C. Bone. St. Louis: Mosby, 1997.

Raeburn, P. and G. DeGeorge. 1997. "You Bet I Mind If You Smoke." *Business Week*, 15 September 1997.

Rau, J. L., Jr. *Respiratory Care Pharmacology*. St. Louis: Mosby, 1994.

Robinson, R. W. and C. W. Zwillich. "Hypoventilation, Central Apnea, and Disordered Breathing Patterns." In *Pulmonary and Critical Care Medicine*, edited by R. C. Bone. St. Louis: Mosby, 1996.

APPENDIX

FINDING OUT MORE

INFORMATION BY PHONE

American Lung Association
1-800-LUNG USA
  This line connects you to the local chapter of this national organization. Obtain information and order literature twenty-four hours a day. Business hours are Monday through Friday 9 A.M. to 5 P.M.

Lung Line
1-800-222-LUNG
  Managed by the National Jewish Medical and Research Center. Registered nurses are available Monday through

Friday, 8 A.M. to 5 P.M. mountain time. Recorded information on common lung diseases is available twenty-four hours a day.

REFERRAL CENTERS

National Jewish Medical and Research Center
Address: 1400 Jackson Street
            Denver, CO 80206
Phone: 1-800-222-LUNG
Internet: http://www.njc.org

A world-renowned medical center for research, evaluation, and treatment of pulmonary diseases (including pulmonary rehabilitation). Patients of any age may be evaluated either as inpatients (if they need urgent hospital care) or as outpatients. Emphasis is placed on patient education and self-monitoring, as well as incorporating family members into patient-support mechanism. Some local hotels offer discounts for patients being treated at the center.

The Alfred I. duPont Institute
duPont Hospital for Children
Address: 1600 Rockland Road
            Wilmington, DE 19899
Phone: (302) 651-4000
Fax: (302) 651-5838

Comprehensive program for children with severe asthma, as well as clinical treatment, research, and medical training for the management of childhood scoliosis.

PULMONARY REHABILITATION CENTERS

Most major hospitals now have rehabilitation facilities. The following are outstanding rehabilitation centers with which I have had direct contact.

Burke Rehabilitation Hospital
Address: 785 Mamaroneck Road
            White Plains, NY 10605
Phone: (914) 948-0050
Fax: (914) 421-0790
  Provides both inpatient and outpatient pulmonary rehabilitation, as well as patient support groups. Patients must not have used tobacco products for three months before they are considered for entry into the programs.

The Pulmonary Rehabilitation Program at
Cheshire Medical Center
Address: 590 Court Street
            Keene, NH 03431
Phone: (603) 352-4111
Fax: (603) 355-2341
Internet: http://www.cheshire-med.com/programs/pulrehab/rehab.html
  Offers comprehensive seven-week outpatient program for patients with chronic lung disease, including complete preprogram evaluation.

Helen Hayes Hospital
Address: Route 9W
            West Haverstraw, NY 10993
Phone: 1-888-70-REHAB
Fax: (914) 947-3087
Internet: http://www.helenhayeshospital.org
  A leading specialty hospital that offers individualized inpatient and outpatient cardiopulmonary rehabilitation.

New York University-Rusk Institute—
Cardiac Prevention & Rehabilitation Center
Address: 550 First Avenue
               New York, NY 10016
Phone: (212) 263-6129
Fax: (212) 263-7476

World-renowned center offering individualized inpatient and out-patient pulmonary rehabilitation program.

St. Francis Hospital—The Heart Center
The DeMatteis Center
Address: 225 Valentine Lane
               Old Brookville, NY 11545
Phone: (516) 629-2435
Fax: (516) 629-2141
Internet: http://www.Stfrancisheartcenter.com/preventive/
               pulmonary.html

Offers complete pulmonary evaluation followed by individualized outpatient program (up to twelve weeks, depending on patient's needs).

NATIONAL SOCIETIES

Allergy and Asthma Network/Mothers of Asthmatics, Inc. (AAN/MA)
Address: 2751 Prosperity Avenue, Suite 150
               Fairfax, VA 22031
Phone: 1-800-878-4403
Fax: (703) 352-4354
Internet: http://www.aaanma.org

Provides accurate, up-to-date information for patients and their families to offer a greater understanding of allergy and asthma. Membership includes subscription to the monthly newsletter "The MA Report," as well as discounts on allergy and asthma products and publications. List of publications, videos, and other informative materials provided by this organization may be obtained by calling the above number.

American Academy of Allergy and Immunology

Address: 611 East Wells Street
Milwaukee, WI 53202
Phone: (414) 272-6071
Fax: (414) 272-6070
Internet: http://www.aaaai.org

Professional society of allergists and related specialists. Publishes *Asthma and Allergy Advocate* for patients and the *Journal of Allergy and Clinical Immunology* for physicians. Educational pamphlets and brochures may be purchased via fax or mail.

American College of Allergy and Immunology

Address: 85 West Algonquin Road, Suite 550
Arlington Heights, IL 60005
Phone: (847) 427-1200
Fax: (847) 427-1294
Internet: http://allergy.mcg.edu/

Professional society of allergists and related specialists. Publishes *Annals of Allergy and Immunology* for physicians. Maintains a web site with information and news service for patients and news media.

American Dietetic Association (ADA)

Address: 216 West Jackson Boulevard
Chicago, IL 60606-6995
Phone: (312) 899-0040
Fax: (312) 899-1979
Internet: http://www.eatright.org

The ADA and its National Center for Nutrition and Dietetics provide nutrition resources and the latest information on nutritional health.

American Lung Association (ALA)

Address: 1740 Broadway
               New York, NY 10019-4374
Phone: (212) 315-8700
Fax: (212) 265-5642
Internet: http://www.lungusa.org

An informative national organization with local chapters throughout the United States. Publishes numerous pamphlets and booklets (see below) on all types of lung disease, as well as audiovisual aids, posters, and signs. ALA also sponsors programs for the lay public on lung disease, smoking cessation, and support groups, as well as asthma camps. One important function of the ALA is to raise funds and sponsor research into lung diseases. Locate your local chapter by calling 1-800-LUNG-USA.

American Thoracic Society (ATS)

Address: 1740 Broadway
               New York, NY 10019-4374
Phone: (212) 315-8700
Fax: (212) 315-6498
Internet: http://www.thoracic.org

The medical branch of the American Lung Association. Besides many scientific activities, ATS/ALA has initiated the Asthma Research Campaign, designed to promote multidisciplinary research aimed at producing a major advance in the prevention and treatment of asthma. ATS also publishes *American Journal of Respiratory and Critical Care Medicine*.

Asthma and Allergy Foundation of America (AAFA)

Address: 1125 15th Street NW, Suite 502
               Washington, DC 2005
Phone: (202) 466-7643
Fax: (202) 466-8940
Internet: http://www.aafa.org

National organization sponsoring educational programs for patients with asthma and allergies. AAFA promotes research and asthma support groups and publishes the newsletter "Advance."

National Asthma Campaign
Address: Providence House
Providence Place
London, N1 ONT
United Kingdom
Phone: 44-171-226-2260
Fax: 44-171-704-0740
Internet: http://www.efanet.org

UK organization comparable to the American Lung Association, with branches throughout the UK. Member of European Federation of Asthma and Allergy Associations.

National Cystic Fibrosis Foundation
Address: 6931 Arlington Road
Bethesda, MD 20814
Phone: 1-800-344-4823
Fax: (301) 951-6378
Internet: http://www.cff.org

National organization for cystic fibrosis.

National Heart, Lung, and Blood Institute (NHLBI)
Address: Information Center
P. O. Box 30105
Bethesda, MD 20824-0105
Phone: (301) 251-1222

The branch of the National Institutes of Health that sponsors cardiovascular and respiratory research and educational activities. Publications for the general public include health information for women and how to stop smoking.

National Institutes of Health (NIH)
Address: 9000 Rockville Pike
              Bethesda, MD 20892
Phone: (301) 496-4000
Internet: http://www.nih.gov

The U.S. government's major center for health research. Web site links to its twenty-four institutes, including the National Library of Medicine.

National Sarcoidosis Resource Center
Address: P. O. Box 1593
              Piscataway, NJ 08855-1593
Phone: (732) 699-0733
Fax: (732) 699-0882
Internet: http://www.nsrc-global.net

Worldwide source of information on sarcoidosis, with a resource guide and directory. Internet site provides links to other sarcoidosis web sites.

NEWSLETTERS

Air Currents
Publisher: Glaxo Wellcome, Inc.
Address: P. O. Box 5875
              Hauppauge, NY 11788
Phone: 1-800-732-7390

Reports on trends in asthma, as well as general information on respiratory disease.

Asthma and Allergy Advocate
Publisher: American Academy of Allergy and Immunology
Address: 611 East Wells Street
              Milwaukee, WI 53202

Phone: (414) 272-6071
    Contains practical advice for patients with asthma and allergies.

Harvard Women's Health Watch
Publisher: Harvard Medical School Health Publications Group
Address: 164 Longwood Avenue
    Boston, MA 02115
Phone: 1-800-829-5921
    Informative monthly publication with current medical information.

Health & Nutrition Letter
Publisher: Tufts University
Address: P. O. Box 57875
    Boulder, CO 80322-7857
Phone: 1-800-274-7581
    General nutritional information and special dietary advice.

The MA Report
Publisher: Asthma and Allergy Network (AAN)/
    Mothers of Asthmatics, Inc.
Address: 2751 Prosperity Avenue, Suite 150
    Fairfax, VA 22031
Phone: 1-800-878-4403
    Published monthly with practical information for families of children with asthma. Patients or parents may write in questions, which are answered by a team of specialists.

New Directions
Publisher: National Jewish Medical and Research Center
Address: 1400 Jackson Street
    Denver, CO 80206
Phone: 1-800-222-LUNG
    Informative publication focused on new developments in respiratory disease.

PERF Second Wind

Publisher: Pulmonary Education and Research Foundation
Address: P. O. Box 1133
              Lomita, CA 90717-5133
Phone: (310) 539-8390

Pulmonary rehabilitation information by one of the field's leading organizations.

BOOKS

American Dietetic Association's Complete Food & Nutrition Guide

Author: Roberta Larson Duyff
Publisher: Chronimed Publishing
Length: 640 pages

Comprehensive guide to foods, nutrition, and diets.

Asthma and Exercise

Authors: Nancy Hogshead and Gerald S. Couzens
Publisher: Henry Holt & Co.
Length: 214 pages

Detailed recommendations for children and adults with asthma on exercise and participation in athletics.

The Asthma Sourcebook

Author: Francis V. Adams, M.D.
Publisher: Lowell House
Length: 206 pages

Everything you need to know about asthma.

Breathing Disorders: Your Complete Exercise Guide

Author: Neil F. Gordon, M.D.
Publisher: Human Kinetics Publishing
Length: 130 pages

The Cooper Clinic and Research Institute fitness series.

Children with Asthma: A Manual for Parents
Author: Thomas Plaut, M.D.
Publisher: Pedipress, Inc.
Length: 268 pages
   Highly comprehensive; valuable for parents of asthmatic children.

Choices
Authors: Marion Morra and Eve Potts
Publisher: Avon Books
Length: 921 pages
   Leading cancer reference guide for consumers, with state-by-state listing of cancer-related organizations and services.

Cystic Fibrosis: The Facts
Authors: Ann Harris and Maurice Super
Publisher: Oxford University Press
Length: 144 pages
   Informative book on all aspects of cystic fibrosis.

Merck Manual: Home Edition
Authors: Berkow, Beers, Fletcher, eds.
Publisher: Merck & Co.
Length: 1,536 pages
   Comprehensive medical reference book. Written in a straightforward style providing medical information from anatomy to drugs.

Shortness of Breath: A Guide to Better Living and Breathing
Author: Andrew L. Ries, ed.
Publisher: Mosby-Year Book
Length: 128 pages
   Provides COPD patients with information on how to cope with their disease.

The Stop Smoking Workbook
Authors: Lori Stevic-Rust and Anita Maximin
Publisher: Fine Communications
Length: 171 pages
    Comprehensive guide to help you stop smoking.

BOOKLETS

The Asthma Handbook (ALA #4002)
(Spanish version (ALA #4003)
Publisher: American Lung Association
Address: 1740 Broadway
        New York, NY 10019-4374
Phone: 1-800-LUNG-USA
    A concise, helpful twenty-four page handbook for adult patients
with asthma.

The Asthma Organizer
Author: Nancy Sanders
Publisher: Allergy and Asthma Network/Mothers of Asthmatics, Inc.
Address: 2751 Prosperity Avenue, Suite 150
        Fairfax, VA 22031
Phone: 1-800-878-4403
    Informative notebook for planning a daily strategy for managing and
monitoring asthma. (Available in Spanish and English.)

Around the Clock with COPD (ALA #1230)
Publisher: American Lung Association
Address: 1740 Broadway
        New York, NY 10019-4374
Phone: 1-800-LUNG-USA
    Prepared with the help of actual COPD patients offering their ideas
and suggestions of how to adjust and enjoy life. This thirty page booklet
is a must for anyone with COPD.

Help Yourself to Better Breathing (ALA #4001)
Publisher: American Lung Association
Address: 1740 Broadway
            New York, NY 10019-4374
Phone: 1-800-LUNG-USA
    A thirty-eight page booklet that explains how you can help yourself
to live your life by breathing better.

Being Close
Publisher: National Jewish Medical and Research Center
Address: 1400 Jackson Street, Room G206
            Lung Line Information Service
            Denver, CO 80206
Phone: 1-800-222-LUNG
    Addresses sexual concerns of patients with respiratory disease.

PAMPHLETS

Fact Sheets
Publisher: American Lung Association
Address: 1740 Broadway
            New York, NY 10019-4374
Phone: 1-800-LUNG-USA
    AAT Deficiency–Related Emphysema (ALA #0426)
    Air Pollution Tips for Exercisers (ALA #0560)
    Asthma (ALA #0052)*
    Chronic Bronchitis (ALA #0139)
    Cigarette Smoking (ALA #0171)
    Emphysema (ALA #0301)
    Home Control of Allergies and Asthma (ALA #3512)
    Lung Cancer (ALA #1282)*
    Nicotine Addiction and Cigarettes (ALA #0182)
    Occupational Asthma (ALA #0211C)
    Peak Flow Meters (ALA #0427)

Pulmonary Fibrosis and Interstitial Disease (ALA #3734)
Sarcoidosis (ALA #0049)
Secondhand Smoke (ALA #1091)*
Tuberculosis (ALA #1091)
        *Available in Spanish

Sneezeless Landscaping
Publisher: ALA of California
Address: 424 Pendleton Way
               Oakland, CA 94621
Phone: (510) 638-8984
    Describes plants that may cause allergic reactions, offers alternatives for your garden.

AUDIOVISUAL AIDS

Aerobics for Asthmatics
Publisher: Aerobics for Asthmatics, Inc.
Address: 10301 Georgia Avenue, Suite 306
               Silver Springs, MD 20902
    Exercise video designed by swimmer and Olympic gold medalist Nancy Hogshead, in cooperation with Stanley I. Wolf, M.D., and Kathy L. Lampl, M.D. Available through Allergy and Asthma Network/ Mothers of Asthmatics, Inc.

Allergy Control Begins at Home
Publisher: Allergy Control Products, Inc.
Address: 96 Danbury Road
               Ridgefield, CT 06866
Telephone: 1-800-422-Dust
Fax: (203) 431-8963
Internet: www.allergycontrol.com
    Informative video containing detailed scientific discussion of the biology and living habits of dust mites, as well as steps to reduce expo-

sure. Includes commentary by experts from the Asthma and Allergic Diseases Center at the University of Virginia.

Sit and Be Fit Exercise Videotapes

Publisher: Sit and Be Fit, Inc.

Address: P. O. Box 8033

           Spokane, WA 99203-0033

Telephone: (509) 448-9438

Fax: (509) 448-5078

    Separate videos for specific physical conditions including *Chronic Obstructive Pulmonary Disease (COPD)* and *Osteoporosis*. Led by Mary Ann Wilson, a registered nurse and star of PBS's *Sit and Be Fit* television programs, the tapes feature stretching, toning, and situation-specific moves. COPD video teaches chest expansion, postural muscles, and diaphragmatic breathing. The osteoporosis video shows postural muscle–strengthening techniques.

ALLERGY AND RESPIRATORY CARE SUPPLIES

Allergy Asthma Technology, Ltd.

Address: 8224 Lehigh Avenue

          Morton Grove, IL 60053

Phone: 1-800-621-5545

Fax: (847) 966-3068

Internet: http://www.allergyasthmatech.com

    Offers a wide selection of allergy and asthma products, with links to allergy and asthma sites. The mail-order catalog includes a wide selection of products to "allergy proof" your home, as well as self-help books and a form for insurance or tax deductions.

Allergy Control Products, Inc.
Address: 96 Danbury Road
              Ridgefield, CT 06877
Phone: 1-800-422-DUST
Fax: (203) 431-8963
Internet: http://www.allergycontrol.com
   A mail-order company providing a large selection of allergy and asthma products. The catalog includes washable stuffed animals.

Lincare
Address: 19337 U.S. 19 North, Suite 500
              Clearwater, FL 34624
Phone: (813) 530-7700
Fax: (813) 532-9692
Internet: http://www.lincare.com
   Respiratory care company with 303 offices in forty-two states. Provides all forms of respiratory care, including oxygen, nebulizers, respirators, and CPAP. Web site provides information on these services, as well as breathing exercises and a general-health newsletter.

ON THE INTERNET: FAVORITE WEB SITES

Allergy and Respiratory Supplies

Allergy Asthma Technology, Ltd.
http://www.allergyasthmatech.com

Allergy Control Products, Inc.
http://www.allergycontrol.com

Lincare
http://www.lincare.com

General Health Information

The Asthma Sourcebook
http://home.earthlink.net/~francisva
Everything you need to know about asthma on-line. This site's Health Watch News page provides current information on asthma, including new FDA-approved medications.

Cheshire Medical Center
http://www.cheshire-med.com
Wide selection of health information with links to numerous health-resource sites. This site has an extensive section on lung disease.

Enact
http://www.enact.com
Introduces you to AirWatch, an electronic peak flow meter that allows you to download this information for your physician.

European Federation of Asthma and Allergy Associations
http://www.efanet.org
Provides information on asthma and allergy, as well as links to European web sites.

Glaxo Wellcome-Asthma Control Program
http://www.asthmacontrol.com
Information from major pharmaceutical companies on how to control your asthma, including "Air Currents" newsletter. You can request a free kit that describes the Asthma Control Program.

Harvard Health Publications
http://www.countway.med.harvard.edu/publications/Health_Publications
This site allows you to sample the five health newsletters that are published by Harvard Medical School.

Mayo Oasis

http://www.mayohealth.org

Health information from the Mayo clinic from cancer and diet to nutrition. This site offers a subscription to *Housecall*, a free weekly web newsletter.

Mental Health-Stress

http://www.teachhealth.com

Offers information on the medical basis of stress, depression, anxiety, sleep problems, and drug use, with amusing graphics and links to both mental- and general-health sites.

New York University Health System

http://www.med.nyu.edu

Award-winning site that includes links to the NYU Medical Center, Rusk Institute of Rehabilitation, and NYU Medical School, among many others.

Sarcoidosis Research Institute

http://www.netten.net/~soskelnt

Information for individuals with sarcoidosis. This site includes a poetry corner and offers links to related Internet locations.

SleepNet

http://www.sleepnet.com

Information on sleep apnea and other sleep disorders.

National Societies

Allergy and Asthma Network/Mothers of Asthmatics

http://www.aanma.org

American Academy of Allergy Asthma & Immunology

http://www.aaaai.org

American Cancer Society
http://www.cancer.org
Information on specific cancers and therapies, with links to other cancer sites. Local ACS can be located through this site.

American Heart Association
http://www.amhrt.org
Heart and stroke A–Z guide. Nutrition and fitness information, with recommendations for reducing risk of heart disease.

American Lung Association
http://www.lungusa.org
Comprehensive information on lung diseases, air quality, and ALA programs. You may register for on-line newsletters, make a donation, or become an ALA volunteer.

Association for Child Psychoanalysis
http://www.westnet.com/acp
International organization whose purpose is to advance the psychological treatment and understanding of children and adolescents and their families.

European Federation of Asthma and Allergy Associations
http://www.efanet.org
An alliance of twenty-seven organizations in fourteen European countries.

Health Care Financing Administration
http://www.hcfa.gov
Medicare and Medicaid Agency, with links to government agencies, including Social Security.

National Institutes of Health
http://www.nih.gov

Home page of NIH provides links to its twenty-four institutes and centers that include National Heart, Lung, and Blood Institute (NHLBI), and National Institute of Allergy and Infectious Diseases.

National Jewish Medical and Research Center
http://www.njc.org

National Women's Health Information Center
http://www.4woman.org
Information about issues and programs affecting women's health, with links to many sites containing women's health related material.

Prescription Medications

Pharmaceutical Information Network
http://www.pharminfo.com
Drug information, with links to drug and disease discussion groups and various science bulletins.

RXList–Internet Drug Index
http://www.rxlist.com
Easy-to-use site to research medications, with links to numerous health-related sites.

SEARCH ENGINES

Ability Index and Search
http://www.ability.org.uk/home.html
Extensive list of disability- and health-related sites, including ones for scoliosis and mental health.

Healthfinder

http://www.healthfinder.gov

U.S. government search engine for Department of Health and Human Services information.

Yahoo

http://www.yahoo.com

Popular search engine with vast health and medicine listings.

GLOSSARY

Acaracide: Agent that kills mites; could be used in the home to eradicate dust mites.

Acetylcholine: Chemical substance stored in nerve endings of parasympathetic nervous system; released when nerves are stimulated, producing a response.

Adenocarcinoma: A malignant tumor that forms a glandlike pattern; the most common type of lung cancer.

Adrenaline: Potent hormone produced by the adrenal gland, with many total-body effects, including the opening (dilatation) of the bronchial tubes. The beta-adrenergic bronchodilators are all derived from adrenaline (epinephrine).

Adrenergic: Refers to sympathetic nervous system and its nerve fibers and receptors.

Aerophagia: Swallowing of air.

Aerosol: Fine mist that can be inhaled; may be produced by metered-dose inhaler or nebulizer.

Agonist: Drug or agent with an affinity for corresponding nerve receptor that may stimulate the receptor to produce its effect.

Allergen: Substance producing allergic reaction.

Allergy: Hypersensitivity to specific substance.

Alveoli: Tiny air sacs that comprise lung tissue where the exchange of oxygen and carbon dioxide occurs.

Alveolitis: Inflammation of the alveoli.

Anaphylaxis: Severe, total-body allergic reaction often characterized by "closing" of the throat and constriction of the bronchial tubes; may result in collapse of the body's circulation (shock), and death.

Angiogram: X-ray of blood vessels after the injection of a dye.

Antibody: Protein substance formed by the body in response to a material (antigen) that stimulates the immune system.

Anticholinergic: Antagonistic to the action of cholinergic or parasympathetic nerves.

Antihistamine: Drug that neutralizes the substance histamine, which is often released in the body during allergic reactions.

Artery: A blood vessel that carries blood away from the heart. With the exception of the pulmonary artery, these vessels contain blood that has been enriched with oxygen.

Atelectasis: Lung condition in which tiny air sacs, or alveoli, are collapsed.

Atopy: Condition of being allergic.

Autonomic nervous system: Involuntary control system that maintains many functions; divided into parasympathetic and sympathetic branches.

Biopsy: Examination of tissue or cells removed from a living patient for the purpose of diagnosis.

Beta-agonist: Medication stimulating nerve receptors that produce bronchial tube dilatation.

Beta-receptor: Nerve-ending site responsible for the bronchial tube condition.

Bronchial tubes: Air passages of the lung through which air exchange takes place.

Bronchiectasis: Condition of the bronchial tubes in which infection damages the wall of the bronchial tube; produces chronic productive cough and recurrent infection.

Bronchioles: The smallest of the bronchial tubes that open into the alveoli.

Bronchoalveolar: Relating to the bronchial tubes and surrounding alveoli; one of the types of lung cancer.

Bronchoconstriction: Narrowing or closing of the bronchial tubes.

Bronchodilatation: Opening or widening of the bronchial tubes.

Bronchodilator: Agent or medication that produces bronchodilatation.

Bronchography: X-ray of the bronchial tubes after injection of dye.

Bronchoscopy: Procedure in which a lighted scope, called a bronchoscope, is introduced into the lungs through the bronchial tubes.

Bronchospasm: Same as bronchoconstriction.

Bullae: A large vesicle or blister.

Cachexia: A general lack of nutrition and wasting occurring in the course of a chronic illness.

Candidiasis: Fungal infection caused by common yeast, called candida.

Capillaries: Tiny blood vessels found in the walls of alveoli in the lungs and other parts of the body.

Carbon dioxide (CO_2): Waste product of body metabolism; gas excreted by the lungs in exhalation.

Carcinoma: A malignant tumor.

Carotid: Pertaining to the carotid artery, which is located in the neck and which contains the body's receptor that senses the blood-oxygen level.

Catheterization: The passage of a tube or catheter; may be used to examine the heart (cardiac catheterization).

Cerebral cortex: The principal part of the brain.

Chemoreceptor: Cells that are stimulated by chemical substances and thus elicit reflex effects.

Cholinergic: Agent or medication stimulating the parasympathetic nervous system.

Cilia: Rodlike extensions of the lining cells of the bronchial tubes; the sweeping motion of the cilia causes mucus to move upward toward the throat, from which it may be expectorated.

Corticosteroid: Group of medications derived from the adrenal gland.

Cyanosis: Dark blue or purplish discoloration of the skin, nail beds, and lips due to a deficiency of oxygen in the blood.

Deconditioned: Lacking physical fitness.

Decongestant: An agent that reduces congestion, usually by constricting the small capillary blood vessels in the nasal passages.

Decubitus: Position of the patient in bed; may also be used to describe a bedsore.

Diaphragm: The large, dome-shaped muscle that divides the chest from the abdomen.

DNA: Abbreviation for deoxyribonucleic acid, the compound that contains the genetic code of living tissue.

Dysphagia: Difficulty swallowing.

Dyspnea: Awareness, difficulty, or distress in breathing.

Edema: The excessive collection of clear, watery fluid in the tissues.

Elastase: An enzyme that works on elastin, a protein found in tissues.

Elastin: The protein substance that is contained in elastic tissue.

Embolectomy: The removal of blood clots.

Embolism: The blockage of a blood vessel by a transported clot or other material.

Empirically: An approach that is based on practical experience but not proven scientifically.

Enzyme: A protein substance that induces a chemical reaction in the body but remains unchanged in the process.

Eosinophil: A type of white blood cell associated with allergic reactions.

Epistaxis: A nosebleed.

Ergometer: Instrument for measuring amount of work or energy the body uses.

Erythema: Redness, inflammation.

Expiratory: Relating to breathing out, or exhaling.

Fibrosis: The formation of fibrous or scar tissue.

Granuloma: A lesion that has a specific form of inflammation, recognizable under the microscope.

Hemoglobin: Protein substance contained in the red blood cell that transports oxygen to the tissues.

Hemoptysis: Blood-spitting.

HEPA: High-efficiency particulate air purifier.

Histamine: Substance produced in the body, which is involved in allergic reactions.

Hyperinflated: Lung condition in which lungs are overexpanded.

Hyperreactivity: Condition of increased sensitivity or irritability, a feature of the bronchial tubes in asthma.

Hypersomnolence: A condition in which one is inclined to sleep at all times.

Idiopathic: Of unknown cause.

Immunoglobulin E: IgE, a type of immunoglobulin produced when a sensitive individual is exposed to allergens.

Immunotherapy: Allergy treatment also known as "desensitization" or "allergy shots." Injections of extracts of allergy substances are given in increasing strengths over time.

Intercostal: Between the ribs.

Intranasal: Refers to application of medication inside nasal passages.

Intravenous: Injecting medication directly into a vein.

Intubation: The placement of a breathing tube into the windpipe, performed when artificial or mechanical ventilation is needed.

Leukotrienes: Substances produced in the body; cause inflammation.

Lobectomy: Surgical removal of individual lobe of the lung.

Lymphatics: Pertaining to vascular channels that connect the lymph glands.

Lymphocyte: White blood cell commonly involved in immune reactions; T lymphocytes are involved in cellular reactions; B lymphocytes produce antibodies.

Mast cells: Body cells that contain chemicals which are mediators of asthma or allergy reactions.

Mechanoreceptor: Receptor that responds to mechanical pressures.

Mediastinum: Central compartment of the chest that contains all the viscera of the chest except the lungs.

Medicamentosa: Relating to a drug.

Mesothelioma: Tumor of the pleura; may be benign or malignant; associated with exposure to asbestos.

Metabolism: The sum of the chemical changes of the body in which nutrients are broken down and used for body functions.

Mucosa: Mucous membrane covering inner surface of many structures of the body, including the nose and bronchial tubes.

Myopathy: Muscle abnormality possibly characterized by weakness and atrophy.

Neuron: A nerve cell.

Neurotransmitter: Chemical substance that facilitates conduction of nerve impulses.

Neutrophil: Type of white blood cell often involved in immune reactions.

Orthopnea: Discomfort on breathing in any but the erect sitting or standing position; usually noted at night when lying down.

Oximeter: Device measuring saturation or enrichment of the blood with oxygen.

Oxygen (O_2): Gas needed for life-sustaining activities of the body; taken up by red blood cells in the walls of the alveoli.

Parasympathetic: Pertaining to a division of the autonomic nervous system.

Paroxysmal: Occurring in paroxysms, or sudden spasms.

Particulates: Fine, airborne particles (soot) produced by fuel combustion; component of air pollution.

Peak flow: The maximum airflow generated with a forced expiration.

Pharynx: The throat.

Phlebitis: Inflammation of a vein.

Phlegm: Mucus.

Pneumonectomy: Surgical removal of an entire lung.

Polypectomy: Surgical procedure to remove polyps from various body locations, including the nose and sinuses.

Protease: A protein-splitting enzyme.

Reflux: Backward flow; term commonly used to describe regurgitation of stomach contents into feeding passage (esophagus).

Rhinoscopy: Inspection of the nose and nasal passages, utilizing a lighted scope (rhinoscope).

Rhinovirus: One of a group of viruses that may cause the common cold.

Rhonchus: A loud, low-pitched, or sonorous chest sound heard with the use of the stethoscope.

Spirometer: Instrument used to measure lung's air capacity; may also be adapted to measure speed of airflow or movement.

Spirometry: Test of pulmonary function, utilizing spirometer.

Sputum: Material coughed from the lungs; also "phlegm," consisting of mucus, cells, and debris resulting from bacteria.

Squamous: Relating to covering cells or tissue; one of the common forms of lung cancer that arises from the lining cells of the bronchial tubes.

Symptomatology: Aggregate of symptoms from disease.

Syncope: Fainting spell.

Systemic: Term referring to the entire body.

Tachycardia: Rapid heartbeat.

Tachypnea: Rapid breathing.

Thorax: The chest cavity.

Thromboembolism: Embolism from a clot dislodged from a blood vessel.

Thrombophlebitis: Inflammation of a vein with clot formation.

Thrombus: A clot in a blood vessel.

Trachea: Main air passage, or windpipe, beginning below the voice box (larynx); divides into right and left main bronchial tubes.

Urticaria: Skin eruption of hives.

Uvula: Soft conelike projection from the soft palate.

Vagus: Major nerve with parasympathetic (cholinergic) nerve fibers distributed to the bronchial tubes; stimulating these nerves may cause constriction. Anticholinergic medications that block vagal impulses may be bronchodilators.

Varicose: Large and tortuous; often used to describe veins.

Vasculitis: Inflammation of blood vessels.

Virus: Term for a group of organisms capable of causing disease in many hosts, including man. Viruses are smaller than bacteria and are only capable of growth within living cells.

INDEX